Engineering Cyber-Physical Systems and Critical Infrastructures 8

Series Editor

Fatos Xhafa, *Departament de Ciències de la Computació, Technical University of Catalonia, Barcelona, Spain*

The aim of this book series is to present state of the art studies, research and best engineering practices, real-world applications and real-world case studies for the risks, security, and reliability of critical infrastructure systems and Cyber-Physical Systems. Volumes of this book series will cover modelling, analysis, frameworks, digital twin simulations of risks, failures and vulnerabilities of cyber critical infrastructures as well as will provide ICT approaches to ensure protection and avoid disruption of vital fields such as economy, utility supplies networks, telecommunications, transports, etc. in the everyday life of citizens. The intertwine of cyber and real nature of critical infrastructures will be analyzed and challenges of risks, security, and reliability of critical infrastructure systems will be revealed. Computational intelligence provided by sensing and processing through the whole spectrum of Cloud-to-thing continuum technologies will be the basis for real-time detection of risks, threats, anomalies, etc. in cyber critical infrastructures and will prompt for human and automated protection actions. Finally, studies and recommendations to policy makers, managers, local and governmental administrations and global international organizations will be sought.

Alireza Souri · Salaheddine Bendak
Editors

Artificial Intelligence for Internet of Things (IoT) and Health Systems Operability

AI for IoT and Health Systems

Springer

Editors
Alireza Souri
Department of Software Engineering
Haliç University
Istanbul, Türkiye

Salaheddine Bendak
Department of Industrial Engineering
Haliç University
Istanbul, Türkiye

ISSN 2731-5002 ISSN 2731-5010 (electronic)
Engineering Cyber-Physical Systems and Critical Infrastructures
ISBN 978-3-031-52786-9 ISBN 978-3-031-52787-6 (eBook)
https://doi.org/10.1007/978-3-031-52787-6

This Springer imprint is published by the registered company Springer Nature Switzerland AG
The registered company address is: Gewerbestrasse 11, 6330 Cham, Switzerland

Paper in this product is recyclable.

Preface

IoTHIC-2023 is a multidisciplinary, peer-reviewed the International Conference on Internet of Things (IoT) used in all fields of health, including health indicators, predicting, and detecting diseases in hospitals, clinics, healthy lifestyle, smart health monitoring systems, occupational injuries, public health, ambulance services, surgery, medical services, traffic injuries, etc. The IoTHIC-2023 has provided a forum for the exchange of the latest technical information using artificial intelligence (AI) techniques such as data mining, machine learning, image processing, and meta-heuristic algorithms. The new paradigm of AI-based techniques has optimized the high-quality research results and presentation of new development case studies in IoT applications. Participants in IoTHIC-2023 came from a wide range of disciplines, including medicine, software engineering, statistics, communication, robot surgery, database specialists, biomedical engineering, cybersecurity, computer engineering, health management, management information systems, electrical engineering, industrial engineering, physics, operations research, mathematics, simulation, occupational safety, and many other fields.

This proceeding contains full research papers and empirical case studies. All received paper submissions were subjected to a technical peer-reviewed process involving expert and independent reviewers. In total, 36 manuscripts were submitted to the conference. Each was reviewed by two reviewers who were external or members of the conference scientific committee members. Fourteen peer-reviewed papers were accepted with an acceptance rate of 38%.

The conference had three technical sessions including Internet of things (IoT) applications in healthcare systems, AI-based techniques, and methodologies on medical systems such as image processing, machine learning, and deep learning, and finally optimization algorithms for health management in hospitals, clinical systems, and health centers.

Accepted papers were presented by one author and discussed with attendants, chair session, and program committee members to identify the main weaknesses, advantages, and future opportunities of each presented paper.

Also, four expert keynote speakers were invited to address IoTHIC-2023 audience. Prof. Dr. Issam El Naqa from Moffitt Cancer Center, Florida, USA, spoke on "Towards trustworthy AI in healthcare." Associate Prof. Dr. Muhammed Ali Aydın from Istanbul University-Cerrahpaşa, Türkiye, talked on "Cyber-Security in Internet of Medical Things (IoMT)." The third keynote speaker, Prof. Dr. Ata Murat Kaynar from the University of Pittsburgh-School of Medicine, Michigan, USA, spoke on "TeleHealth in Turkey and Beyond: Access, Equity, Equality, and Environment." Finally, Dr. Gabriella Casalino from the University of Bari, Italy, talked on "Digital Healthcare for Internet of Medical Things (IoMT)."

The authors would like to thank Ms. Şeyda Yoncaci for helping in editing this book. Thanks for collaborating with all attendees, authors, members of conference committees, and session chairs. Special thanks are given to the Rector of Halic University

Prof. Dr. Zafer Utlu as the Honorary Chair of IoTHIC-2023, for providing continuous support throughout the preparations process.

October 2023

Alireza Souri
Salaheddine Bendak

Organization

Honorary Chair

Zafer Utlu	Haliç University, Türkiye

General Chairs

Alireza Souri	Haliç University, Türkiye
Salaheddine Bendak	Haliç University, Türkiye
Salaheddine Bendak	Haliç University, Türkiye
Alireza Souri	Haliç University, Türkiye

Organizing Committee

Salaheddine Bendak	Haliç University, Türkiye
Alireza Souri	Haliç University, Türkiye
Figen Özen	Haliç University, Türkiye

Advisory Committee

Cem Alhan	Acıbadem Maslak Hospital, Türkiye
Mu-Yen Chen	National Cheng Kung University, Taiwan
Gwanggil Jeon	Incheon National University, Korea
Ata Murat Kaynar	University of Pittsburgh, USA
Michal Grivna	University of the United Arab Emirates, UAE
Mingliang Gao	Shandong University of Technology, China
Muhammed Ali Aydın	Istanbul University-Cerrahpaşa, Türkiye
Alessandro Calvi	Università Degli Studi Roma Tre, Italy
Eyhab Al-Masri	University of Washington, USA
Gabriella Casalino	University of Bari, Italy
Elif Altıntaş Kahriman	Haliç University, Türkiye
Iffat Elbarazi	University of the United Arab Emirates, UAE

Contents

Drug-Drug Interaction, Interaction Type and Resulting Severity Forecasting by Machine Learning-Based Approaches

Muhammed Erkan Karabekmez[1](✉), Arafat Salih Aydıner[2], and Ahmet Şener[3]

[1] Department of Bioengineering, Istanbul Medeniyet University, Istanbul, Turkey
erkan.karabekmez@medeniyet.edu.tr
[2] Department of Management, Istanbul Medeniyet University, Istanbul, Turkey
[3] Institute of Graduate Studies, Department of Biological Data Science, Istanbul Medeniyet University, Istanbul, Turkey

Abstract. Drug-drug interactions can be discovered by wet-lab experiments. Considering huge amount of possible drug combinations, knowing the drugs that are likely to interact before starting these scientific investigations will provide great savings in terms of time, labor and cost. In this study, it is aimed to identify the best machine learning algorithm to detect not only unknown drug-drug interactions but also to assign type and severity of the predicted interactions. We have applied the molecular structure of drugs, their targets, classification codes, and enzyme effects as inputs and tested logistic regression, naive bayes, K-nearest neighbor, decision trees and deep learning methods. The best performance was attained by deep neural networks (DNN). 88% average success rate has been reached by cross training of the DNN model. The lowest success rates were received for test sets including many severe interactions. Our study demonstrates that DNN can predict not only potential drug-drug interactions but also whether the interaction type is pharmacokinetics or pharmacodynamics. Our model differentiates minor and moderate interaction severities fairly but weak in differentiating severe interactions because of small number of known severe interactions in the training set.

Keywords: Drug-Drug Interaction · Deep Learning · Artificial Intelligence · Adverse Drug Reactions

1 Introduction

Unwanted Drug-Drug interactions (DDI) can lead to severe side effects, adverse reactions, poisoning and even death (Edwards and Aronson 2000). DDIs cause a significant increase in healthcare costs (Jha et al., 2001) as they are one of the most common causes of adverse drug reaction (ADR). Three to six percent of ADRs in hospitalization process is reported to be caused by DDIs (Leape et al., 1995). Various computational methods have been developed to predict drug pairs that may interact with each other. Basically, there are three types of methods in estimating drug-drug interactions. These are methods developed based on the similarities of drugs, methods developed using networks, and methods using machine learning algorithms (Qiu et al., 2021).

A. Souri and S. Bendak (Eds.): IoTHIC 2023, ECPSCI 8, pp. 1–11, 2024.
https://doi.org/10.1007/978-3-031-52787-6_1

Drug-drug interactions (DDIs) are one of the most common causes of adverse drug reaction (ADRs), and these symptoms have been reported to be common in the elderly using multiple drugs (Gallelli et al., 2002). ADRs represent a common clinical problem and may be responsible for the increased number of hospitalizations and/or length of stay (Lee et al., 2000). When use of multiple drugs causes an ADR and this is evaluated incorrectly, it can cause new drugs to be added to the patient's prescription and trigger new ADRs from DDIs (Rochon and Gurwitz, 1997). Combination of drugs is common practice to increase the effectiveness of drug therapy, but the selection of the optimal combination and optimal doses remains a matter of trial and error. Therefore, the prediction of synergistic, additive, and antagonistic responses to drug combinations in vivo remains a highly interesting topic (Jonker et al., 2005).

There are also in vitro assays that are aimed at guiding chemists and biologists in their decision-making processes. The role of these early tests is to indicate obligations in scaffolds regarding the absorption, distribution, metabolism and cytochrome P450 (CYP) inhibition potential of new chemical entities. Bioanalytical method development in DDI screening is divided into four basic categories: strategies for enzyme kinetics, recognition of CYP variants, and creation of computational models to predict CYP interactions (Hutzler et al., 2005).

Supervised Machine Learning (SML) is the search for algorithms that reason from externally provided examples to generate general hypotheses and then make predictions about future examples. Supervised classification is one of the most frequently performed tasks by intelligent systems (Friedman, 2006; Osisanwo et al., 2017). As the supervised basic machine learning algorithms that are more interested in classification, we can list the following: Linear Regression, Logistic Regression, Naive Bayes Classifier, Support Vector Machines, Decision Trees, Random Forest Classifier, Artificial Neural Networks Bayes Networks, etc. (Ayodele, 2010).

Knowledge-based methods such as topological analysis, matrix factorization, logistic regression, Naïve Bayes networks, decision trees, K-nearest neighbors, support vector machines, label propagation, Bayesian probability model, shortest path length average, deep learning networks, deep feed-forward networks and graph convolutional networks were used to predict drug-drug interactions in the literature (Angermueller et al., 2016; Ayodele, 2010; Friedman, 2006; Osisanwo et al., 2017; Samuel et al., 1959; Vilar et al., 2012).

There are many studies in the literature trying to predict ADRs. Tatonetti et al. (2012) manually identified eight groups of phenotypes of clinical significance. For each phenotype, they trained the output with the Logistic Regression method (Tatonetti et al., 2012). Vilar et al. (2012) took into account only structural similarities (Vilar et al., 2012). Gottlieb et al. (2012) calculated different similarities of drug pairs accounting for chemical similarity, ligand-based chemical similarity, similarities based on registered and predicted side effects, the Anatomical Therapeutic Chemical (ATC) classification system, sequence similarity, distance over protein-protein interaction (PPI) network, and Gene Ontology (GO) similarities (Gottlieb et al., 2012). In the system developed by Cheng and Zhao (2014), ATC classification codes, chemical structure similarities, genomic structure similarities, and phenotypic similarities that cause ADR are calculated and used in multiple computational approaches (Cheng and Zhao, 2014). Huang et al. (2013) conducted a network learning study to find pharmacodynamic drug-drug interactions (Huang et al., 2013). Park et al. (2015) conducted a study on finding pharmacodynamic interactions based on the assumption that the effect of two drugs on the same gene would change the effectiveness of the drugs (Park et al., 2015). Qian et al. (2019) showed that the targets of negatively interacting drugs tend to have more synergistic genetic interactions than the targets of non-interacting drugs (Qian et al., 2019). In another study, Deng et al. (2020) used Graph neural networks to capture topological structure information and semantic relationships of drugs (Deng et al., 2020). In their study, Mei and Zhang (2021) constructed a protein-protein interaction network and a network of protein pathways. They then applied a logistic regression model to measure the interaction intensity, interaction effectiveness, and range of effects between the two drugs by summing up the results (Mei and Zhang, 2021). Feng et al. (2020) do not take any properties related to drugs as input in their study. This has enabled the model to be used in cases where some drug properties are missing (Feng et al., 2020).

Finally, all these prior studies showed that there is no model that determines the interaction of drug pharmacokinetics and pharmacodynamics. In addition, a method that predicts drug interactions in terms of severity has not been tested yet.

In this study, firstly, the data will be taken and stored in a structural and relational way. Then, required cleaning will be done in order to use this data in machine learning and transformation processes. Estimation models will be tested and the most appropriate method will be determined.

2 Materials and Methods

2.1 Collecting and Structuring Data

The data we used in our study were taken from the Drugbank database (version 5.1.8 released on January 3, 2021). In the Drugbank database, there are more than two hundred properties of each drug, as well as information about the interaction of drugs with each other (Wishart et al., 2018). 2,706 approved small molecule drugs, 1,505 approved biologicals (proteins, peptides, vaccines, and allergenics), 132 nutraceuticals, and over 6,655 experimental molecules (discovery phases) are covered in the Drugbank. The data was downloaded in XML format.

Python programming language was used to extract the data from the XML file and load it into the relational database system. The structural database that we parse the data from the XML file and put it is Oracle XE 21c version. With Oracle XE, 12 GB of data and 2 GB of memory are free to use.

The resulting DRUG table contains general information about drugs such as drug name, drug description, drug type, drug properties. The DRUGBANK_ID field in this table is the primary key of the table and holds a unique code number for each drug.

The DRUG_PAIRS table holds information about the drug pairs interacting with each other and explanations about how this interaction is. The interaction types of drugs (pharmacokinetic, pharmacodynamics) and the severity of the interactions of drugs, as well as the similarity of the molecular structures of the drugs were calculated and added to this table. The DRUG_TARGET table contains the target information of the drugs, and the DRUG_ENZYMES table contains the enzyme information for the drugs. The

DRUG_ATC_CODES table also contains the ATC classification code information of the drugs. 167-bit MACCS molecule vectors created by using Simplified Molecular-Input Line-Entry System (SMILES) (Weininger 1988). The codes of drugs are placed in the DRUG_MACCS table. The enzyme information on which drugs act has been added to the DRUG_ENZYME_VECTOR table by turning it into a vector. A total of 458 enzyme information is kept in this table for each drug.

There is a total of 14,315 drug information in the Drugbank database. Out of these, drugs that are approved and in the form of small molecules (molecular weight less than 900 daltons) were filtered. Then proteins and drugs used on the outer surface of the body (creams and ointments) were excluded. Lastly, the drugs with missing information were also excluded and remaining 650 drugs were selected for the study.

For the selected drugs there are 210,925 combinations for potential interactions. Known interactions and interaction types of these drug pairs are given in Table 1.

Table 1. Distribution of drug-drug interaction types and severity

-		Number of Interactions
Interaction Type	Pharmacokinetic	37,708
	Pharmacodynamic	41,790
Severity	Minor Impact	20,186
	Medium Impact	58,176
	Major Impact	1,140
Total		79,498

Tanimoto Coefficient (Tanimoto 1958) was used to calculate similarity scores between molecular pairs based on their SMILES codes. We make use of the Rdkit library (Landrum, 2013) in python for transforming chemical structures into vector format.

The DNN structure for this research was created with the Keras library in the python programming language. The DNN structure we created with Keras has a total of 6 layers, including 1 input layer, 1 output layer and 4 intermediate layers. The input layer receives 1280 input information and transmits it to the middle layers. The middle layers have 128, 64, 64, 64 nodes respectively. Finally, the output layer has 3 output nodes, and each node outputs a probability number.

3 Results

The Tanimoto Coefficients were calculated for each drug pair covered and recorded as a similarity matrix. The Drugbank bank brought 1300 values for each drug. Subjecting so many features to the learning process in machine learning models leads to excessive learning problems. To get rid of this, feature reduction methods have been applied. Key Components Analysis (KCA) was used after standardization to reduce the number of data to be used in the models. A 50-valued vector was obtained for each drug using this method. Both standardized and non-standardized datasets were tested.

Drugs can be classified in a single or multiple Anatomical Therapeutic Chemical (ATC) category. This requires an arrangement of ATC codes. A vector was prepared with a classification code (0 or 1) for each ATC category. The length of the resulting ATC vector was 712. This number was reduced to 50 by using PCA in order to prevent excessive learning problems.

Another vector was created for representing enzyme and target data in order to account for interactions with CYP enzymes which may activate or inhibit metabolism of other drugs (Srinivas et al., 2017). Again, PCA was used to reduce the size of the vector. To apply machine learning techniques, various transformations to the four vectors for each drug carrying above mentioned properties were implemented, resulting in different variations. We prepared 8 different vectors as input to machine learning algorithms to see which vector transforms work better together. These data sets include 4 properties of drugs as well as drug-drug interaction information that we pulled from Drugbank. The format of the data to be submitted into the model with these arrangements were consisting of similarity vector of drug A (with respect to drug B), similarity vector of drug B (with respect to drug A), ATC code vector of drug A, ATC code vector of drug B, enzyme vector of drug A, enzyme vector of drug B, target vector of drug A, the target vector of drug B, interaction types and severity. The content of the eight datasets were presented in Table 2.

Ryu et al. (2018) tried the similarity vector of drugs with PCA method with 10, 20, 30, 40 and 50 columns and got the best result for 50 columns. In our study, we tried vectors as 50 columns and 100 columns. In addition, we tried the whole vector set to measure the success of the models.

For data training, Logistic Regression (LR), Naive Bayes (NB), Decision Trees (DT), K-Nearest Neighborhood (K-NN), and Deep Learning Networks (DLN) were applied to the same data separately. 90% of the total data is included in the training, while 10% is reserved for tests. F1-scores were calculated to determine performance for the applied data with the test data and are shown in Table 3. It is seen that DLN provides a superior success compared to other methods in predicting drug-drug interactions.

In the next step, with the same data sets, this time it was tried to predict not only the drug-drug interactions, but also the type of interaction (pharmacokinetic or pharmacodynamic) and the severity of the interaction (minor, moderate or major). To make this possible, the last layer of the neural network is labeled with 7 different values Table 4. For example, number 0 means that there is no interaction between two drugs, number 3 means that there will be an interaction between drugs, this type of interaction will be pharmacokinetic, and the degree of severity is 3 etc.

After deep neural networks are trained with given inputs, the performance of learning is measured with test data. As a result of the estimation with deep neural networks, we get an output that gives the probability of each tag being present. This always equals 1 when we add up the probability of all labels. So, when we make an estimation in our model, we will have 7 probability values in total for 7 label types. While calculating the performance of the model, the label with the highest probability is taken as the output. Then, this value is compared with the actual label value, and a performance score is obtained. The success scores of the machine learning methods in finding only DDI showed that the most successful method is DLN.

Table 2. Contents of data sets to be tested in models

	D1	D2	D3	D4	D5	D6	D7	D8
Similarity Vector 50	✔	✔						
Similarity Vector 50 Std.					✔			
Similarity Vector 100 Std.				✔				
Similarity Vector 100			✔					
Similarity Vector – All						✔		
Enzyme-Vector (CYP)	✔	✔	✔	✔	✔	✔		
Enzyme Vector – All							✔	✔
Target Vector – All	✔							
Target Vector 50		✔	✔					✔
Target Vector 50 Std				✔	✔	✔	✔	✔
Interaction Information	✔	✔	✔	✔	✔	✔	✔	✔
Pharmacokinetic Information	✔	✔	✔	✔	✔	✔	✔	✔
Pharmacodynamic Information	✔	✔	✔	✔	✔	✔	✔	✔
Severity Information	✔	✔	✔	✔	✔	✔	✔	✔

Table 3. F1-Scores of data sets in predicting interactions

	LR	NB	DT	K-NN	DLN
Data Set 1	0.78	0.43	0.85	0.82	0.92
Data Set 2	0.75	0.57	0.86	0.83	0.90
Data Set 3	0.91	0.56	0.84	0.82	0.90
Data Set 4	0.75	0.55	0.84	0.79	0.88
Data Set 5	0.74	0.54	0.85	0.79	0.85
Data Set 6	0.79	0.64	0.83	0.79	0.82
Data Set 7	0.73	0.51	0.85	0.79	0.83
Data Set 8	0.76	0.42	0.86	0.83	0.90
Average	0.7763	0.5275	0.8475	0.8063	0.875

To test the 7 categories determined by deep neural networks, our machine learning model was arranged to have 7 outputs. Then the model was run and its performance was examined. In order to increase the model performance, new experiments were made by changing the number of layers and nodes in the model. To solve the over-learning problem, the efficiency of some nodes has been reduced. As a result, the solution with the highest performance and closest to the optimum was determined. This solution was applied to the 8 datasets we have.

Table 4. Generating DLN output labels

#Class	Pharmacokinetic Interaction	Pharmacodynamic Interaction	Severity	Tag
0	0	0	0	0
1	1	0	1	101
2	1	0	2	102
3	1	0	3	103
4	0	1	1	11
5	0	1	2	12
6	0	1	3	13

Cross-validation helps us to understand whether the performance achieved is random or is it really achievable. Our model was tested with the 10-fold cross-validation method and its performance were tested. In the previous validation test, 90% of the data was set for training and 10% for testing. In the cross-validation process, we repeated the same test 10 times with different training and test sets. We calculated the actual performance of the model by averaging the F1 scores each time. Figure 1 shows how the training and test data were selected. Equation 1 shows how the average performance is calculated.

$$performance = \frac{1}{10}\sum_{i=1}^{10} F1 - score_i \quad (1)$$

When the DNN structure we prepared for 8 different data sets was run and 10-fold cross-validation was performed, the performance results can be seen in Table 5. In the established deep learning network model, the first data set gave the best results and produced an F1 score of 0.861. When the results are examined carefully, a general decrease in success is observed in the 4th, 5th, 6th and 7th iterations. To find out the reason for this, we looked more closely at the distributions in the iterations. When the test data distributions for each iteration are examined, we see that the distributions of classes 3 and 6 in Table 5 are more distributed over the test data in these iterations. In these distributions, both classes 3 and 6 are of major interaction severity, that is, interactions that cause very significant effects.

In other words, in these iterations, drug relations, which are considered to be major in severity, could not be successfully captured in the deep learning network. Although 86% is considered successful, the low prediction success of a feature with a small sample size makes us think that the deep learning model cannot serve its purpose. The confusion matrices showed that there was no positive prediction at all for this feature.

Deep learning networks were trained to predict the features other than severity fairly. When classes containing only interaction types were selected the results of the training and subsequent tests brought 2% improvement on average (Table 6). Data 1 attained the highest performance score.

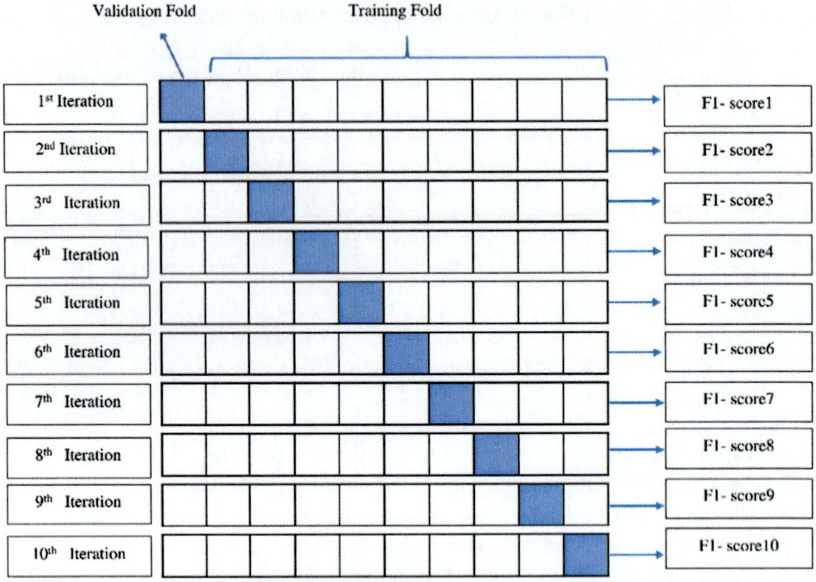

Fig. 1. Selection of Training and Test Data for 10-fold Cross Validation

Table 5. Deep learning network cross validation results

Iteration	D1	D2	D3	D4	D5	D6	D7	D8
1	0.93	0.92	0.92	0.89	0.89	0.90	0.87	0.92
2	0.92	0.90	0.91	0.88	0.87	0.88	0.85	0.90
3	0.92	0.91	0.92	0.89	0.89	0.89	0.87	0.91
4	0.78	0.73	0.74	0.66	0.66	0.67	0.60	0.74
5	0.72	0.64	0.65	0.56	0.55	0.59	0.48	0.66
6	0.72	0.64	0.66	0.54	0.50	0.53	0.46	0.65
7	0.72	0.64	0.66	0.60	0.56	0.59	0.56	0.65
8	0.98	0.98	0.98	0.98	0.97	0.97	0.96	0.98
9	0.98	0.98	0.98	0.97	0.97	0.96	0.96	0.97
10	0.94	0.93	0.93	0.92	0.91	0.91	0.89	0.93
Average	0.861	0.827	0.835	0.789	0.777	0.789	0.75	0.831

Table 6. Deep learning network cross validation results (interaction types only)

Iteration	D1	D2	D3	D4	D5	D6	D7	D8
1	0.95	0.93	0.94	0.90	0.90	0.91	0.88	0.93
2	0.94	0.91	0.92	0.89	0.86	0.88	0.85	0.92
3	0.94	0.92	0.93	0.90	0.89	0.90	0.85	0.93
4	0.80	0.76	0.78	0.70	0.69	0.70	0.64	0.76
5	0.78	0.70	0.73	0.63	0.61	0.65	0.61	0.72
6	0.76	0.69	0.74	0.60	0.58	0.60	0.54	0.71
7	0.73	0.67	0.69	0.60	0.59	0.62	0.59	0.70
8	0.98	0.98	0.98	0.96	0.97	0.94	0.95	0.98
9	0.98	0.98	0.98	0.97	0.96	0.95	0.95	0.97
10	0.95	0.94	0.94	0.91	0.91	0.90	0.89	0.93
Average	0.881	0.848	0.863	0.806	0.796	0.805	0.775	0.855

4 Conclusion

When DDI's cannot be detected beforehand and interacting drug pairs are given to the patients, it can cause severe results. In this study, we created a prediction model by applying machine learning methods to predict drug-drug interactions. We tested logistic regression, naive bayes, K-nearest neighbor, decision trees and deep learning methods on our data to reach the most appropriate result. We have advanced our model in this direction, seeing that the most efficient result is obtained when deep learning networks are used.

In this study, for the first time, we studied a model that predicts the type of interaction of drugs, namely whether there is a pharmacokinetic or pharmacodynamic interaction, and the severity of the interaction.

Our models were successful in predicting interaction type whereas were not satisfactory for severity prediction. Main reason for this is the small number of high-severity samples in the dataset.

As a result of training the models, we achieved a success rate of 73% to 98%, with an average of 88%, according to the sample set in our most efficient model. Cheng and Zhao (2014), who made drug interaction estimation with similar input data, achieved a 67% success rate by using SVM by calculating the similarity profiles of drugs. In the method proposed by Ryu et al. (2018), training with DNN using only the similarity profiles of drugs showed a success of 92.4% for 86 different interaction types. Lee et al. (2019), who developed this model, included the structural similarity profile of drug targets and gene ontology data with the feed-forward DNN model and included it in the model and carried this success rate to 97%.

Our results presented at Table 6 and 7 shows that best results came with 50 column non-standardized inputs. Together with the information in Table 2, it can be proposed as a further work to inclusion of all-enzyme and all-target data together with 50 column non-standardized similarity data can improve the presented results. As the datasets in Drugbank or similar database will get mature by filling missing information, larger and more reliable training datasets will be beneficial in not only predicting the DDI's but also their type and severity of the interactions.

References

Angermueller, C., Pärnamaa, T., Parts, L., Stegle, O.: Deep learning for computational biology. Mol. Syst. Biol. **12**(7), 878 (2016)

Ayodele, T.O.: Types of machine learning algorithms. New Adv. Mach. Learn **3**, 19–48 (2010)

Cheng, F., Zhao, Z.: Machine learning-based prediction of drug-drug interactions by integrating drug phenotypic, therapeutic, chemical, and genomic properties. J. Am. Med. Inf. Assoc. JAMIA **21**(e2), e278–e286 (2014). https://doi.org/10.1136/amiajnl-2013-002512

Deng, Y., Xu, X., Qiu, Y., Xia, J., Zhang, W., Liu, S.: A multimodal deep learning framework for predicting drug–drug interaction events. Bioinformatics **36**(15), 4316–4322 (2020)

Edwards, I.R., Aronson, J.K.: Adverse drug reactions: definitions, diagnosis, and management. Lancet **356**(9237), 1255–1259 (2000)

Feng, Y.H., Zhang, S.W., Shi, J.Y.: DPDDI: a deep predictor for drug-drug interactions. BMC Bioinf. **21**(1), 1–15 (2020)

Friedman, J.H.: Recent advances in predictive (machine) learning. J. Classif. **23**, 175–197 (2006)

Gallelli, L., et al.: Adverse drug reactions to antibiotics observed in two pulmonology divisions of Catanzaro, Italy: a six-year retrospective study. Pharmacol. Res. **46**(5), 395–400 (2002)

Gottlieb, A., Stein, G.Y., Oron, Y., Ruppin, E., Sharan, R.: INDI: a computational framework for inferring drug interactions and their associated recommendations. Mol. Syst. Biol. **8**, 592 (2012). https://doi.org/10.1038/msb.2012.26

Huang, J., Niu, C., Green, C.D., Yang, L., Mei, H., Han, J.D.: Systematic prediction of pharmacodynamic drug-drug interactions through protein-protein-interaction network. PLoS Comput. Biol. **9**(3), e1002998 (2013). https://doi.org/10.1371/journal.pcbi.1002998

Hutzler, M.J., Messing, D.M., Wienkers, L.C.: Predicting drug-drug interactions in drug discovery: where are we now and where are we going? Curr. Opin. Drug Discov. Devel. **8**(1), 51–58 (2005)

Jonker, D.M., Visser, S.A., van der Graaf, P.H., Voskuyl, R.A., Danhof, M.: Towards a mechanism-based analysis of pharmacodynamic drug-drug interactions in vivo. Pharmacol. Ther. **106**(1), 1–18 (2005)

Jha, A.K., Kuperman, G.J., Rittenberg, E., Teich, J.M., Bates, D.W.: Identifying hospital admissions due to adverse drug events using a computer-based monitor. Pharmacoepidemiol. Drug Saf. **10**(2), 113–119 (2001)

Landrum, G.: Rdkit documentation. Release 1 1–79, 4 (2013)

Leape, L.L., et al.: Systems analysis of adverse drug events. JAMA **274**(1), 35–43 (1995)

Lee, C.E., et al.: The incidence of antimicrobial allergies in hospitalized patients: implications regarding prescribing patterns and emerging bacterial resistance. Arch. Intern. Med. **160**(18), 2819–2822 (2000)

Lee, G., Park, C., Ahn, J.: Novel deep learning model for more accurate prediction of drug-drug interaction effects. BMC Bioinf. **20**(1), 415 (2019). https://doi.org/10.1186/s12859-019-3013-0

Mei, S., Zhang, K.: A machine learning framework for predicting drug–drug interactions. Sci. Rep. **11**(1), 17619 (2021)

Osisanwo, F.Y., Akinsola, J.E.T., Awodele, O., Hinmikaiye, J.O., Olakanmi, O., Akinjobi, J.: Supervised machine learning algorithms: classification and comparison. Int. J. Comput. Trends Technol. (IJCTT) **48**(3), 128–138 (2017)

Park, K., Kim, D., Ha, S., Lee, D.: Predicting pharmacodynamic drug-drug interactions through signaling propagation interference on protein-protein interaction networks. PLoS ONE **10**(10), e0140816 (2015). https://doi.org/10.1371/journal.pone.0140816

Qian, S., Liang, S., Yu, H.: Leveraging genetic interactions for adverse drug-drug interaction prediction. PLoS Comput. Biol. **15**(5), e1007068 (2019)

Qiu, Y., Zhang, Y., Deng, Y., Liu, S., Zhang, W.: A comprehensive review of computational methods for drug-drug interaction detection. IEEE/ACM Trans. Comput. Biol. Bioinf. **19**(4), 1968–1985 (2021)

Rochon, P.A., Gurwitz, J.H.: Optimising drug treatment for elderly people: the prescribing cascade. BMJ **315**, 1096–1099 (1997)

Ryu, J.Y., Kim, H.U., Lee, S.Y.: Deep learning improves prediction of drug-drug and drug-food interactions. Proc. Natl. Acad. Sci. U.S.A. **115**(18), E4304–E4311 (2018). https://doi.org/10.1073/pnas.1803294115

Samuel, A.L.: Some studies in machine learning using the game of checkers. IBM J. Res. Dev. **3**(3), 210–229 (1959). https://doi.org/10.1147/rd.33.0210

Srinivas, M., Thirumaleswara, G., Pratima, S.: Cytochrome P450 enzymes, drug transporters and their role in pharmacokinetic drug-drug interactions of xenobiotics: a comprehensive review. Peertechz J. Med. Chem. Res. **3**(1), 001–011 (2017)

Tanimoto, T. T. (1958). Elementary mathematical theory of classification and prediction

Tatonetti, N.P., Fernald, G.H., Altman, R.B.: A novel signal detection algorithm for identifying hidden drug-drug interactions in adverse event reports. J. Am. Med. Inf. Assoc. JAMIA **19**(1), 79–85 (2012). https://doi.org/10.1136/amiajnl-2011-000214

Vapnik, V. (1999). The nature of statistical learning theory. Springer science & business media

Vilar, S., Harpaz, R., Uriarte, E., Santana, L., Rabadan, R., Friedman, C.: Drug-drug interaction through molecular structure similarity analysis. J. Am. Med. Inf. Assoc. JAMIA **19**(6), 1066–1074 (2012). https://doi.org/10.1136/amiajnl-2012-000935

Weininger, D.: SMILES, a chemical language and information system. 1. Introduction to methodology and encoding rules. J. Chem. Inf. Comput. Sci. **28**(1), 31–36 (1988)

Wishart, D.S., et al.: DrugBank 5.0: a major update to the DrugBank database for 2018. Nucleic Acids Res. **46**(D1), D1074–D1082 (2018)

Hybrid Network Protocol Information Collection and Dissemination in IoT Healthcare

Asaad Adil Shareef and Hasan Abdulkader(✉)

Electrical and Computer Engineering, Altinbas University, Istanbul, Turkey
203720048@ogr.altinbas.edu.tr, Hasan.abdulkader@altinbas.edu.tr

Abstract. In recent years, the internet of things (IoT) has grown in significance, affecting a larger variety of areas of daily life in a wider number of nations. As a result, there has to be a trustworthy system for collecting and disseminating data sent online by trillions of sensors to trillions of actuators. Only a few healthcare scenarios necessitate the transmission of data in real time; in most cases, monitoring relies on the average of sensor readings. Real-time transmission is seldom ever necessary in healthcare applications. Constrained Application Protocol (CoAP) and Message Queuing Telemetry Transport (MQTT) are the two most popular application layer protocols utilized by low-resource devices and Internet of Things applications. However, this study created an architecture that combines MQTT's quick availability with CoAP's dependable and fundamental communication to increase healthcare's reliability and efficiency. Whether the control server uses MQTT or CoAP for message exchange depends on how important the object being controlled is. MQTT protocol proposes several advantages over CoAP such as reliability, real time transmission, broadcasting to topics' subscribers etc. The combination of both MQTT and CoAP allows to filter the health data into two categories, severe symptoms measurements of emergency are published and diffused via brokers using MQTT while normal measurements are conveyed to normal servers using CoAP.

Keywords: Hybrid network protocol · Information collection · Dissemination · IoT healthcare · Real application

1 Introduction

In the world of computers and networking, a concept known as the "Internet of Things" (IoT) is one that will fundamentally alter the landscape. It refers to the practice of giving everyday objects network connectivity in order to enable them to collect and exchange data through the internet [1]. The number of devices that are linked to the internet has increased at a rate that has never been seen before, and it is anticipated that this pattern will continue to expand at an exponential rate until the year 2023 [1].

A. Souri and S. Bendak (Eds.): IoTHIC 2023, ECPSCI 8, pp. 12–27, 2024.
https://doi.org/10.1007/978-3-031-52787-6_2

In the modern world, Internet of Things (IoT) devices may be located virtually anywhere, including homes, companies, vehicles, and even airplanes. Machine-to-machine communication, also known as M2M communication [2] is utilized by these devices in order to collect data in real time through the use of sensors, microcontrollers, and network connections. After then, the information is stored on the cloud, which makes it possible for more advanced system features and intelligence.

The Internet of Things has shown tremendous promise for improving service delivery in the healthcare industry. Patients of all ages may reap the benefits of remote monitoring and improved treatment owing to IoT in healthcare thanks to the collection, processing, and transfer of sensor data to healthcare professionals via networked devices [3]. Patients can profit from IoT in healthcare thanks to enhanced treatment and remote monitoring. Patients now have the option of wearing sensors that are lightweight and tiny to monitor their health. These sensors, in case of emergency, communicate data in real time to medical professionals, allowing for more efficient diagnosis and treatment [1].

The Internet of Things' application in healthcare has been notably beneficial in poor countries where access to medical treatment is limited. The Internet of Things has enabled health monitoring equipment to interact with mobile devices, which has resulted in both a decrease in the cost of healthcare and an increase in its availability [4]. It may be possible for doctors to monitor and analyze patient data in real time using mobile computers, which might lead to improved therapy.

The dynamic interaction between digital and physical systems made possible by sensors and actuators is referred to as the "Internet of Things" (IoT) [5]. It gives objects the ability to establish their own networks, share data with one another, and adapt to the environment around them [6]. The Internet of Things (IoT) research is being conducted with the intention of equipping everyday objects with the sensing and communication capabilities necessary for them to assume control of jobs that were previously carried out by humans, such as monitoring, control and decision-making.

The Internet of Things makes use of a wide variety of technologies and protocols in order to simplify the process of connecting devices and exchanging data. Internet Protocol version 6, IEEE 802.15.4, and Internet Protocol version 6 over Low-Power Wireless Personal Area Network (6LoWPAN) are examples of common protocols for device communication [7]. It is necessary to guarantee that data is interoperable and available by making use of web servers or cloud services that come equipped with their own built-in interfaces [8], regardless of the communication protocol that is used.

The Internet of Things (IoT) is expected to be used in a variety of industries, with healthcare being one of the most promising. Internet of Things (IoT) applications in healthcare add to comprehensive healthcare information systems by enhancing monitoring and decision-making [9]. Examples of these applications include medical telehealth, telemedicine, and home healthcare for patients in their homes or during mobility. It is of the highest importance to include wireless sensor networks into healthcare delivery systems in order to enable the transmission of critical clinical data.

The Internet of Things has the ability to connect anything from household appliances to automobiles, which would then enable the automatic collection and transmission of data [10]. This technology enables greater tracking, monitoring, and management by offering essential insights on user behavior and activity levels. These insights may be used to better manage and track user activity. The combination of internet of things and cloud computing makes data transport and access more streamlined, which in turn makes it simpler to carry out routine tasks with increased velocity and precision [11].

The Internet of Things is undergoing a transformative effect on a variety of industries, one of which is healthcare, thanks to its capacity to connect everyday objects to the internet and enable the collection and exchange of data. The Internet of Things has the potential to reduce costs incurred by healthcare providers, improve the level of care provided to patients, and increase the number of people who have access to medical treatment. The integration of Internet of Things technologies with cloud computing opens up far more opportunities than was before possible. In this study, we propose the use of a hybrid network protocol for the collecting and distribution of data on the Internet of Things (IoT) healthcare sector as a means of overcoming the challenges that have been outlined and making healthcare systems more efficient.

The main contribution of this paper is the combination of the protocols MQTT and CoAP in a library in order to offer better management of health data depending on the emergency of the patient situation. Also, we propose practical application of the IoT-based e-health system using Arduino and Raspberry Pi. The realization collects data via the Arduino and communicates the data to the Raspberry Pi which performs data processing and compares the severity of the received signal to predefined thresholds. The Raspberry controls the transmission of the patient's data either via a CoAP protocol in case of ordinary measure or by publishing the data in real time, with high priority to concerned health services medicines.

2 Problem Statemint

The Internet of Things has become a pioneering technological industry that enters all areas of life, including health care. As a result of its expansion, it faces many challenges, the most important of which is that these systems are trustworthy in order to be efficient and maintain information security. The other problem is the real access time for data, which occurs due to network congestion. With a huge amount of data, so we are facing challenges that need serious solutions.

Among IoT protocols, namely MQTT and CoAP are interesting and provide high throughput. They also provide important services related to security, compatibility, etc. The presentation of application protocols is given below. CoAP is based on UDP protocol, so it is used for fast transmission via short datagrams without connection guarantee. On the other hand, MQTT protocol is based on TCP messaging, it provides short message exchange with 3 levels of QoS. MQTT is suitable for addressing instantaneous messages to given subscribers, healthcare workers in our case, to raise critical healthcare situations.

3 Application Layer Protocols

The term "Internet of Things" (IoT) refers to the rapid proliferation of networked devices that have profoundly impacted the way in which humans interact with technological systems. Now, anything from sensors and actuators to everyday household appliances can connect with one another, which opens up a whole new universe of opportunities for software and services. The Application Layer is the most important part of this ecosystem since it is responsible for easing communication and interaction in both directions between people and Internet of Things devices. A number of application layer protocols have been established to simplify communication in IoT settings. These protocols were built to satisfy the particular challenges and requirements of IoT settings. In this part, we will talk about the protocols Advanced Message Queuing Protocol (AMQP), Data Distribution Service (DDS), Constrained Application Protocol (CoAP), and Message Queuing Telemetry Transport (MQTT). IoT devices are dependent on these protocols in order to share data in a manner that is both safe and effective. These devices connect the digital and physical worlds. Because of their one-of-a-kind characteristics and capacities, they make it possible for developers to construct highly functioning applications and services for the internet of things.

3.1 AMQP (Advanced Message Queuing Protocol)

AMQP is a well-known message-oriented middleware protocol that ensures reliable and risk-free communication between applications. It functions very well on publish-subscribe networks as well as peer-to-peer ones. As a result of the standardization of AMQP messages, systems written in various languages may be able to function together without a hitch. AMQP is comprised of three basic components: the Exchange, the Queue, and the Binding, each of which is responsible for queuing and traffic management in its own specific way. The protocol's transport layer is responsible for managing errors and providing the framing, while the protocol's function layer is in charge of providing more complex communication capabilities. AMQP frames must adhere to a precise structure that consists of a header and a body, and there are many different types of AMQP frames that are used for a variety of purposes. The protocol is functional with both straightforward messages and those that are more complicated and come with attachments of information. AMQP brings flexibility, interoperability, and dependability to the table when it comes to messaging in IoT systems [12, 13].

3.2 DDS (Data Distribution Service)

The Object Management Group (OMG) has standardized the Data Distribution Service (DDS), which is a Publish-Subscribe protocol that permits exchange of data in nearly real-time. It functions under a broker-less architecture and relies on multicasting for stable communication. Additionally, it was created without a middleman. The Data Distribution Service (DDS) is comprised of two layers: DCPS, which stands for Data-Centric Publish-Subscribe, and DLRL, which stands for Data Local Reconstruction Layer. DCPS is in charge of managing all connections, whereas DLRL is responsible for adding functionality and assisting with the integration of apps. The DDS communication paradigm is comprised of its five key components: Publishers, Data Writers, Subscribers, Data Readers, and Topics. To the Department of Defense assistance Activity, DDS provides assistance for Quality of Service (QoS) requirements in order to assure privacy, responsiveness, priority, sturdiness, and dependability. Real-Time Publish-Subscribe (RTPS), which is based on either UDP/IP or TCP, is the wire protocol that it employs. An RTPS message always includes standard components such a header, one or more body messages, and a conclusion. Using the plugin-based security measures that are offered by DDS, protecting sensitive information is a simple and straightforward process [14].

3.3 COAP (Constrained Application Protocol)

COAP is a protocol for the application layer of the Internet of Things that was created specifically for low-resource devices. It makes it possible to communicate effectively while using fewer resources. The RESTful architecture of COAP offers a number of benefits, including support for multicasting, little overhead, and an easy learning curve for users. It employs the utilization of the UDP protocol, which enables data to expand beyond its initial very small packet size. The asynchronous client-server communication that COAP provides includes all of the following message types: Confirmable, Non-confirmable, Acknowledgement, and Reset. A header structure is utilized by the protocol in order to provide message transfer and functionality related to requests and responses. Requests and responses are two distinct types of COAP communications that may be distinguished by the Method Codes and Response Codes that are associated with them. COAP is compatible with a wide variety of protocols due to the RESTful nature of the protocol [15–17].

3.4 MQTT (Message Queuing Telemetry Transport)

MQTT, a lightweight communications protocol that uses a Publish-Subscribe model, is extremely important to the Internet of Things. It ensures the flow of data reliability while spending very little power, making it ideal for systems with restricted resources. The MQTT architecture includes a server, a client, and a group of subscribers in addition to themselves. Connecting clients will submit inquiries to the servers, while content producers will write to subjects, and readers will sign up to get updates on particular themes. The protocol provides a wide variety of Quality of Service (QoS) levels in order to ensure that messages are sent and received in a timely manner. The binary protocol utilized by MQTT is appropriate for use in real-world applications due to the fact that it has a minimal overhead and experiences a low volume of traffic. I provides the ability to make advantage of its persistent sessions, stored messages, and legacy support. MQTT's ubiquity, ease of usage, and scalability have led to its widespread adoption in Internet of Things deployments [7, 18]. MQTT protocol was used in [19] to convey images captured using YOLO-v4 implemented on IoT devices to detect masked and badly masked people. [20] used the MQTT for remotely monitoring patients in healthcare systems. Authors of [21] used also MQTT to transmit physiological data collected by wearable devices. Wearable devices use Bluetooth communication protocol and conveyed to remote monitoring using the MQTT protocol.

In this paper the combination of the protocols MQTT and CoAP in a library offers better management of health data distribution depending on the severity of the patient situation. The controller connected to IoT devices, analysis the data and swith transmission of the data either through MQTT protocol to inform immediately healthcare workers or by CoAP transmission to an ordinary server for archiving. The practical application illustrated the IoT-based e-health system using Arduino and Raspberry Pi.

The realization collects data via the Arduino and communicates the data to the Raspberry Pi which performs data processing and determines serious situations in received signal. The Raspberry controls the transmission of the patient's data either via a CoAP protocol in case of ordinary measure or by publishing the data in real time, with high priority to concerned health services medicines.

AMQP, DDS, COAP, and MQTT are all examples of application layer protocols, and they each play a significant part in ensuring that the requirements for communication between IoT devices and applications are met. The qualities and advantages of a protocol can guide developers in making the decision that is best for their project on the protocol to use.

4 Proposed Methodology

This study investigated the most widely used standardized protocols for Internet of Things (IoT), such as CoAP and MQTT, as well as their applications in Internet of Things healthcare. This section provides a description of the unified approach, which combines several protocols into a single library, in order to further satisfy the desire for ways that are more successful in tracking an individual's health. The plan takes into account both the pros and cons associated with each protocol in order to design a healthcare monitoring system for the Internet of Things that is capable of utilizing all of the protocols to their full potential.

When it comes to IoT healthcare, it is imperative that medical professionals and caregivers receive quick notifications about any potential issues. However, because to the limitation imposed by set frequencies, it may be challenging for CoAP-attached devices such as Arduinos to communicate data in the most efficient manner. Because of this constraint, sensor data may be lost at low frequencies, while an overload on the database server may occur at high frequencies. The utilization of TCP by MQTT, on the other hand, ensures dependability yet broadcasts every value, despite the fact that the overwhelming majority of them are pointless. By integrating the aforementioned libraries, we will illustrate in the next part a way that takes use of both CoAP and MQTT in the following paragraph.

4.1 CoAP and MQTT Integration

This section will explain how the CoAP and MQTT protocols may be combined within the approach that has been suggested. When a threshold value is determined, the data from the sensors is transmitted immediately to the MQTT broker, where it is stored until it is ready to be relayed via CoAP. After that, the broker immediately tells any and all parties that may be interested, such as the attending physician and any other caregivers. CoAP is employed for the transfer of normal data at a standard frequency in order to maintain the efficiency of the system, whereas MQTT is utilized for the speedy transmission of important threshold values.

4.2 Methodology in Steps

In this section, the recommended approach is broken down into its component parts, with an emphasis placed on the chronological sequence in which these stages take place. After sending CoAP queries, sensor readings are read from Arduinos, the values are wrapped and delivered, and ultimately, they are evaluated based on the thresholds that were set. Other phases involve getting patient information, retrieving local and internet databases, and using CoAP queries to acquire the most recent sensor value. All of these components—the control server, the end devices, the MQTT broker, and the databases—are able to interact with one another in an efficient and unobtrusive manner thanks to this method.

4.3 Implementation/Simulation Tools

The hardware, software, programming languages, and servers used to implement and simulate the suggested technique are discussed in this section.

Hardware.
The Raspberry Pi 3 was employed as the control server, Arduinos were utilized as the end devices, and a variety of sensors, including the DHT22, were utilized in order to measure the ambient conditions. Additionally listed are digital thermometers, blood pressure monitors, and heart rate trackers.

Programming Languages.
Describes the programming languages that were utilized in the implementation, including Python for the command server and the Arduino programming language, which is a simplified version of C/C + +, for the Arduinos.

Software.
Included is an overview of the software stack, beginning with the integrated development environment (IDE) for Python and progressing via the IDE for Arduino to the installation of PHP5 and the MySQL library on the Apache server in order to link the Raspberry Pi to the MySQL database. There is also discussion of using a database management system (DBMS), such as myphpadmin.

Servers.
The myphpadmin database management server and the Apache web server which are both functioning on the Raspberry Pi are highlighted, as are the other servers which are participating in the implementation.

Figure 1, which depicts the system architecture, and Fig. 2, which depicts the sequence diagram, both can be incorporated into the respective subsections so that they can serve as visual representations and make it easier to understand the recommended strategy.

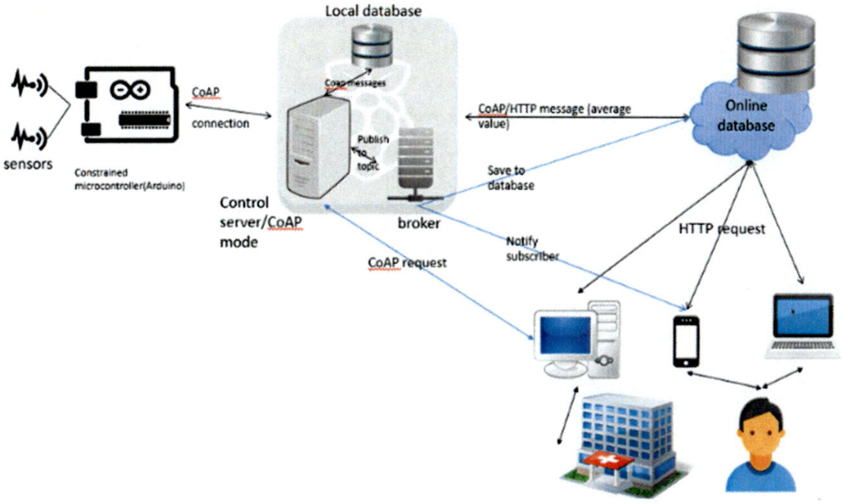

Fig. 1. System Architecture

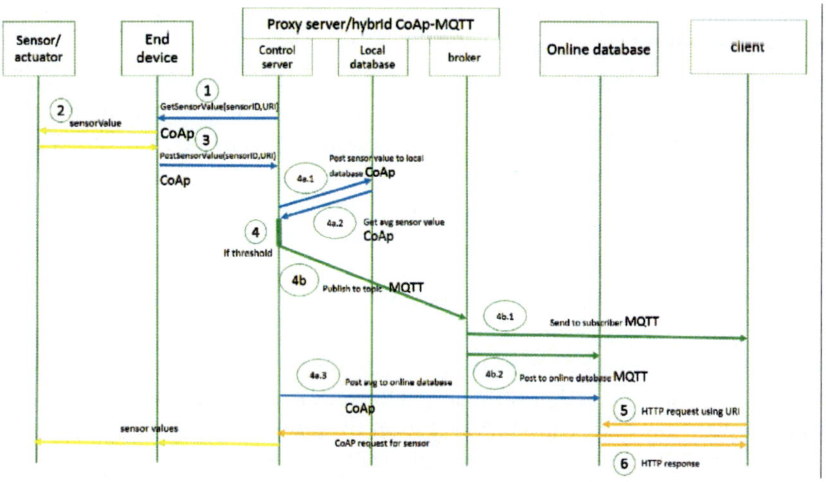

Fig. 2. Sequence diagram

5 Implementation and Results Discussion

The feasibility of the proposed architecture was investigated by employing a Raspberry Pi computer as the control server. CoAP and MQTT are included in a library by means of this approach. The Raspberry Pi, which was given an IP address and linked to a local network in order to fulfill its role as the control server, served as the host for both a neighborhood database and an in-house MQTT broker. By executing a Python script on the Raspberry Pi through the terminal (python server.py), we were able to obtain the behavior of the control server that is displayed in Fig. 3.

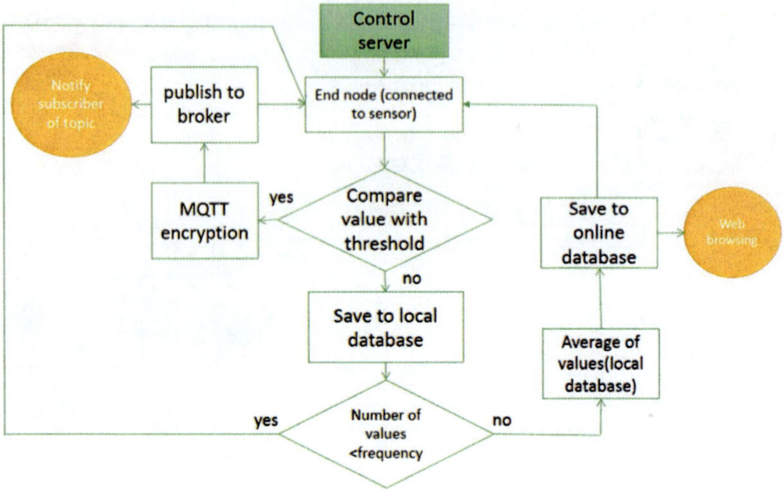

Fig. 3. Flowchart of control server code

After entering the IP address of the Arduino into the Python script, it became possible for the Raspberry Pi and the board to communicate with one another. In an infinite loop, the Raspberry Pi would send CoAP requests to Arduino, which would then poll the Arduino for sensor data at the rate that was specified in the code. In accordance with the requirements outlined in the CoAP standard, the request made a reference to a particular sensor value by using the identification that was assigned to it (sensorID). After then, a CoAP response containing the data gathered from the sensor was sent back to the Raspberry Pi, which acted as the control server. The control server took the value that was included inside the message and compared it to the threshold that was associated with the sensor. Whenever a certain threshold event occurred, denoting the existence of an urgent circumstance, a MQTT message was written, then encrypted, and transmitted to a broker on a topic that had been selected in advance. The data from the sensors that fell within the typical range but did not quite meet the threshold necessary to activate the CoAP frequency were recorded in a local database. After that, a value that was computed using a weighted average of the locally stored variables and transmitted to the cloud. Clients have the ability to acquire a comprehensive report by submitting an HTTP request.

Figure 4 depicts the operations being carried out by a second C++ application that was created for an Arduino. This program follows the techniques indicated above.

Simulations were run to test both the practicability of the solution that was recommended and the compatibility of CoAP with MQTT. Input was provided by a potentiometer that was attached to the Arduino board, and the code was sent to the board using a serial connection (see Fig. 5 for further details). The data was transferred to the organization's online database (depicted in Fig. 6), which is kept on a separate workstation that is connected to a SQL server. The result of the code is displayed in the server's console in Fig. 7, which is also depicted with the potentiometer readings. If the value of the sensor was higher than the threshold, the information was sent to a MQTT broker; otherwise, it was saved in a local database. After a certain number of iterations, the values that make up the local database's average were sent to the remote database. Serial

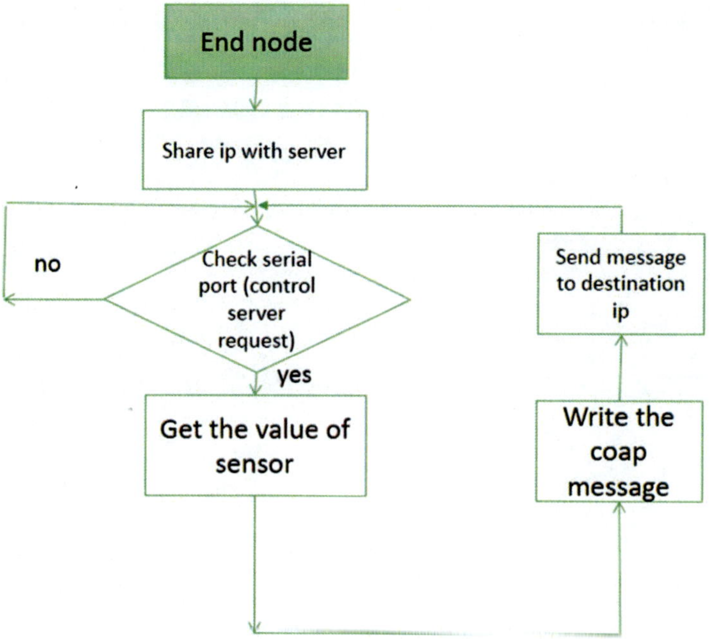

Fig. 4. Flowchart of the Arduino code

communication was used for the CoAP connection between the Arduino and Raspberry Pi (although Wi-Fi with ESP is also an option). This was done so that the process could be kept as straightforward as possible. Figures 9 and 10 illustrate how to access the local database on the Raspberry Pi by using the browser and the localhost/phpMyAdmin URL, as well as how to connect to a remote database by utilizing the IP address of the localhost as the connection point. If the Raspberry Pi merely had the MQTT broker installed, all of the measured values from the publisher (sensor) would be forwarded to the cloud-based database (Figs. 7, 8, 9). This may soon overload both the network and the database. Installing just the CoAP server on the Raspberry Pi might result in the loss of some crucially important measured values since CoAP servers give data at specific intervals as mentioned in the code. By combining the two protocols into a single library, one may make use of all the benefits that each of the protocols offers. The library can connect with the control server through the transmission of a CoAP response message that contains the beginning value. If the value is valid, it will remain in the local storage until the CoAP frequency encourages an average of all the local values to be transmitted to the cloud. If the value is not valid, it will be removed from the local storage. If the result is significantly different from what would be expected, the data is immediately uploaded to the database that is stored in the cloud. If the value is larger than a specific threshold, instead of waiting for the CoAP frequency, the control server will operate as a publisher for the MQTT broker. This will happen if the condition is met. The MQTT broker then sends simultaneous notifications on the patient's critical status to all of the intended subscribers (Fig. 10).

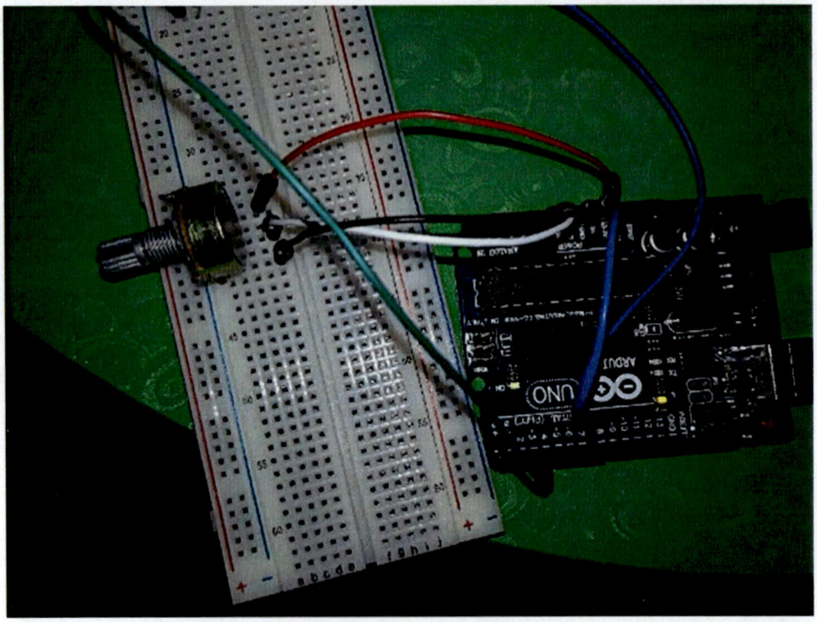

Fig. 5. Implementation of Arduino connected to a potentiometer to test the performance of the system under sensor output variations

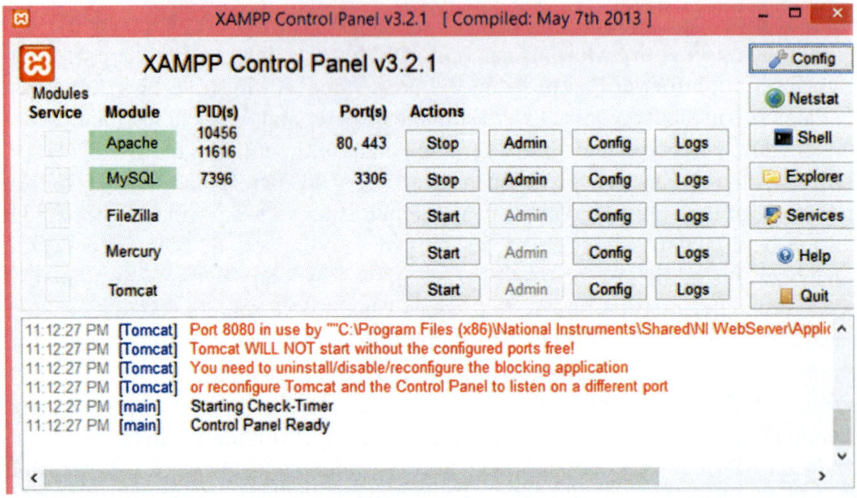

Fig. 6. Run SQL Server

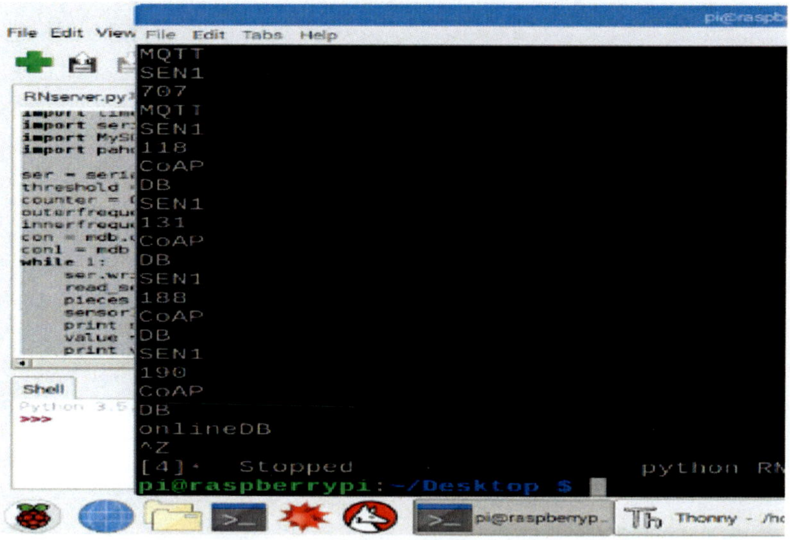

Fig. 7. Terminal of raspberry running new server

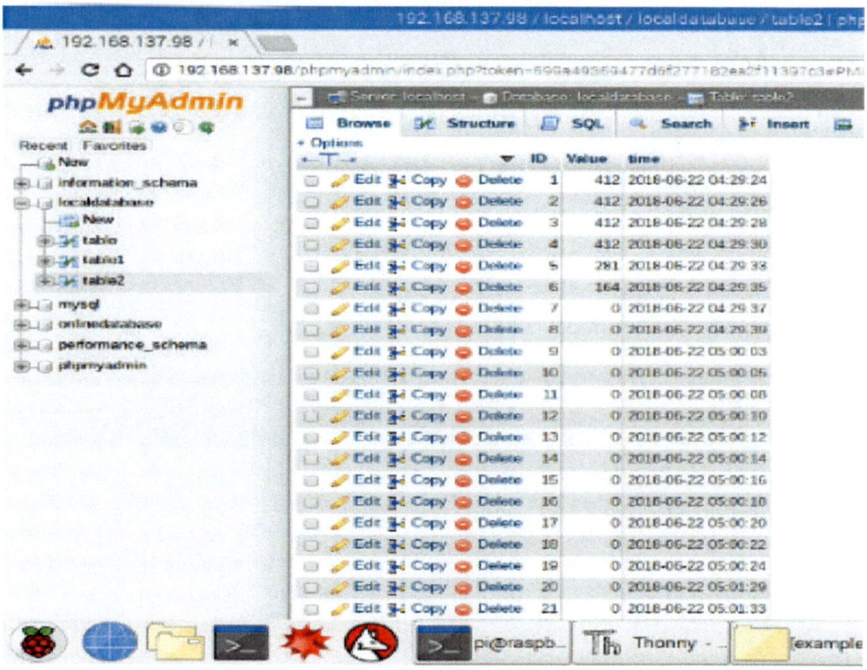

Fig. 8. Local database

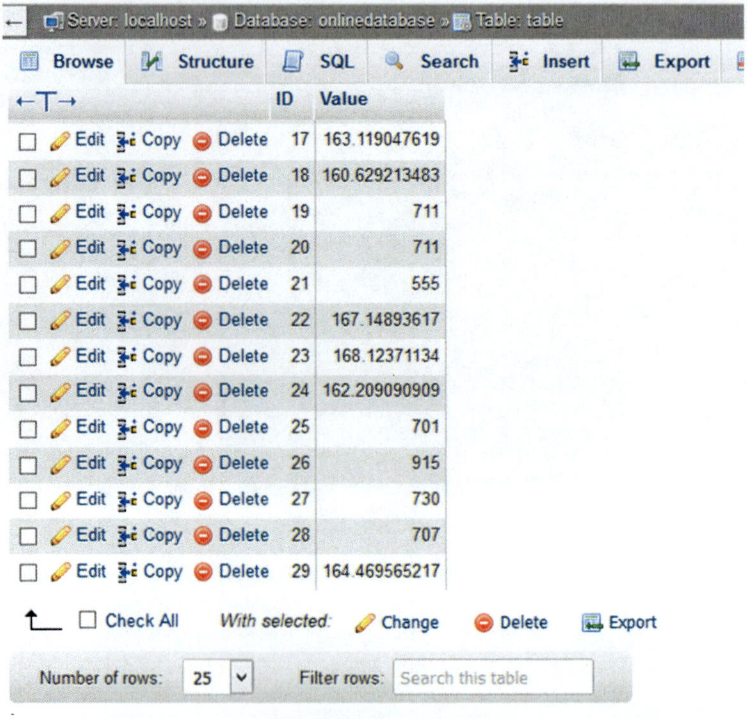

Fig. 9. Online database

T	Sensor value	Ahared on network and stored on database			
		CoAP with frequency 1hz	CoAP with frequency 0.25 hz	MQTT	CoAP/MQTT
1	37	37	37	37	37
2	36.8	36.8		36.8	
3	36.5	36.5		36.5	
4	37	37		37	
5	37	37	37	37	36.825
6	39	39		39	39 MQTT publish
7	37.5	37.5		37.5	
8	37.6	37.6		37.6	
9	37.1	37.1	37.1	37.1	
10	36.9	36.9		36.9	37.275
11	36.9	36.9		36.9	
12	37	37		37	
13	36.7	36.7	36.7	36.7	

Fig. 10. Database Comparison

In conclusion, the integrated library demonstrated its value by demonstrating its capacity to improve the effectiveness of healthcare applications by reducing the strain placed on the networks of healthcare providers and increasing the dependability of the services provided to patients by those providers.

Without losing generality, the actual simulation can be viewed as a model of, among other things, the output of a temperature sensor, a heartbeat sensor, and a blood pressure sensor. In addition, in the situation of many thresholds and multi-sensors, approaches based on machine learning, such as linear regression or multilayer perceptrons, can be used to specify the sampling rate of transmitted measurements. Although ML can provide optimized regression of the sampling rate, simpler look-up table implementation can roughly replace machine learning in the controller to support multiple actions, starting with sending all standard measurements through CoAP protocol, broadcasting samples of the measurements through brokers and MQTT protocol, or broadcasting all measurements in real-time via MQTT protocol if the situation requires it.

In our paper, we considered single threshold case, and by updating the potentiometer position, it produces a range of analog values. In order to detect abnormal values, the controller applied the threshold to the received data. Therefore, the controller switches between MQTT and CoAP protocols depending on the measurements. For values higher than the threshold, the controller invokes MQTT protocol to broadcast real-time measures to caregiving services, while it uses CoAP for measurements below the threshold that are communicated and stored into a dedicated server.

6 Conclusion

Healthcare settings have examined CoAP and MQTT integration. The IoT is affecting organizations across the board, including healthcare, with more connected devices and the need to share data. This necessitates study into resource-constrained device communication methods. MQTT's pub/sub messaging model and reliable communication support outperform CoAP's lightweight and resource-efficient communication, which is preferable for devices with low resources. Using both protocols to better healthcare applications was recommended. A Python-based control server on a Raspberry Pi was installed to handle data translation and processing. We utilized Arduino UNO and ESP8266 Wi-Fi modules to collect sensor data and deliver it to the Raspberry Pi. The control server established a threshold to transform data into CoAP or MQTT messages. CoAP would routinely upload sensor values from the Raspberry Pi to a cloud database. The MQTT broker immediately received sensitive sensor values over the threshold. The simulation results showed that the proposed system can process sensor data, adapt to thresholds, and transfer data to the cloud database and relevant subscribers fast. By integrating the two protocols, which balanced network congestion and reliability, life-threatening patient warnings became achievable. Scalability and performance tracking will determine success. Securely sharing patient health data requires a larger Raspberry Pi network with peer-to-peer connections at each end node. Data rates and RTT between terminals, Raspberry Pi, and cloud database would be beneficial. The recommended library may integrate CoAP and MQTT to provide an effective IoT-based healthcare monitoring system. Picking and combining the best elements of different protocols can reduce network congestion, increase reliability, and simplify crucial messages for patients and healthcare professionals. As the IoT transforms healthcare, this study improves communication solutions.

References

1. Darshan, K.R., Anandakumar, K.R.: A comprehensive review on usage of Internet of Things (IoT) in healthcare system. In: 2015 International Conference on Emerging Research in Electronics, Computer Science and Technology, ICERECT 2015, pp. 132–136 (2016). https://doi.org/10.1109/ERECT.2015.7499001
2. Gillis, A.S.: Internet of Things. https://www.techtarget.com/IoTagenda/definition/Internet-of-Things-IoT. Accessed 19 Dec 2022
3. Gope, P., Hwang, T.: BSN-Care: a secure IoT-based modern healthcare system using body sensor network. IEEE Sens. J. **16**(5), 1368–1376 (2016). https://doi.org/10.1109/JSEN.2015.2502401
4. Dhar, S.K., Bhunia, S.S., Mukherjee, N.: Interference aware scheduling of sensors in IoT enabled health-care monitoring system. In: Proceedings - 4th International Conference on Emerging Applications of Information Technology, EAIT 2014, pp. 152–157 (2014). https://doi.org/10.1109/EAIT.2014.50
5. Kodali, R.K., Swamy, G., Lakshmi, B.: An implementation of IoT for healthcare, 2015 IEEE recent advances in intelligent computational systems. RAICS **2015**, 411–416 (2016). https://doi.org/10.1109/RAICS.2015.7488451
6. HaddadPajouh, H., Dehghantanha, A., Parizi, R.M., Aledhari, M., Karimipour, H.: A survey on internet of things security: requirements, challenges, and solutions. Internet of Things **14**, 100129 (2021). https://doi.org/10.1016/J.IOT.2019.100129
7. Katsikeas, S., et al.: Lightweight & secure industrial IoT communications via the MQ telemetry transport protocol. In: 2017 IEEE Symposium on Computers and Communications (ISCC), Heraklion, Greece, pp. 1193-1200 (2017).https://doi.org/10.1109/ISCC.2017.8024687
8. Gupta, P., Indhra om prabha, M.: A survey of application layer protocols for internet of things. In: Proceedings - International Conference on Communication, Information and Computing Technology, ICCICT 2021 (2021). https://doi.org/10.1109/ICCICT50803.2021.9510140
9. Xia, F., Yang, L.T., Wang, L., Vinel, A.: Internet of Things. Int. J. Commun. Syst. **25**(9), 1101–1102 (2012). https://doi.org/10.1002/DAC.2417
10. Asim, M.: A survey on application layer protocols for internet of things (IoT). Int. J. Adv. Res. Comput. Sci. **8**(3), 996–1000 (2017). https://doi.org/10.26483/IJARCS.V8I3.3143
11. Buyya, R., Broberg, J., Goscinski, A.M. (eds.): Cloud Computing: Principles and Paradigms. John Wiley & Sons, Nashville, TN (2011)
12. Aiyagari, S., et al.: AMQP advanced message queuing protocol protocol specification a general-purpose messaging standard. Tech. Report Version 0–9–1 (2008)
13. OASIS advanced message queuing protocol (AMQP) version 1.0, part 3: messaging. Oasis-open.org. http://docs.oasis-open.org/amqp/core/v1.0/os/amqp-core-messaging-v1.0-os.html. Accessed 13 Sep 2023
14. Rti.com. https://www.rti.com/hubfs/_Collateral/Datasheets/rti-datasheet-connext-dds-pro.pdf. Accessed 13 Sep 2023
15. Khattak, H.A., Ruta, M., Eugenio Di Sciascio, E.: CoAP-based healthcare sensor networks: a survey. In: Proceedings of 2014 11th International Bhurban Conference on Applied Sciences & Technology (IBCAST) Islamabad, Pakistan (2014)
16. Mi, Z., Wei, G.: A CoAP-based smartphone proxy for healthcare with IoT technologies. In: Proceedings of the IEEE International Conference on Software Engineering and Service Sciences, ICSESS, vol. 2018-November, pp. 271–278 (2019). https://doi.org/10.1109/ICSESS.2018.8663785

17. Yadav, R.K., Singh, N., Piyush, P.: Genetic CoCoA++: genetic algorithm based congestion control in CoAP. In: Proceedings of the International Conference on Intelligent Computing and Control Systems, ICICCS 2020, pp. 808–813 (2020). https://doi.org/10.1109/ICICCS48265.2020.9121093
18. Oasis-open.org. http://docs.oasis-open.org/mqtt/mqtt/v3.1.1/errata01/os/mqtt-v3.1.1-errata01-os-complete.doc. Accessed 13 Sep 2023
19. Vu, V.Q., Tran, M.-Q., Amer, M., Khatiwada, M., Sherif, S., Ghoneim, M., Elsisi, M.:. 2023. "A Practical Hybrid IoT Architecture with Deep Learning Technique for Healthcare and Security Applications" Information 14, no. 7: 379. https://doi.org/10.3390/info14070379
20. Hamoud, H.: Alshammari, The internet of things healthcare monitoring system based on MQTT protocol. Alex. Eng. J. **69**, 275–287 (2023). https://doi.org/10.1016/j.aej.2023.01.065
21. Chang, C.-S., Wu, T.-H., Wu, Y.-C., Han. C.-C.: Bluetooth-based healthcare information and medical resource management system. Sensors **23**(12), 5389 (2023). https://doi.org/10.3390/s23125389

CNN-Based Model for Skin Diseases Classification

Asmaa S. Zamil. Altimimi[1] and Hasan Abdulkader[2(✉)]

[1] Electrical and Computer Engineering Department, Altinbas University, Istanbul, Turkey
[2] Engineering Faculty, Halic University, Istanbul, Turkey
hasan.abdulkader@yahoo.com

Abstract. In our daily lives, deep learning (DL) is becoming more and more important. Cancer detection, predictive medicine, autonomous vehicles, weather forecasting, and speech recognition are just some of the commercial uses of AI, it has already made a big impact. As pattern recognition algorithms, classifiers need well designed feature extractors since the performance, overall, depends on the quality of training. This study demonstrates the classification of skin diseases using deep learning and convolutional neural networks with deep layers. However, the proposed model was successful in terms of classification accuracy more than (85.8%) thanks to the increase in layer count, improved feature extraction, and precise selection of kernel sizes for each layer. The suggested approach can divide skin conditions into six groups. To the best of our knowledge, the proposed model outperforms state-of-the-art models; moreover, a significate comparison is presented in this research paper.

Keywords: Skin Diseases · Convolutional Neural Networks · Deep Learning · Image Classification

1 Introduction

Skin diseases are more prevalent than other diseases. Skin diseases can be caused by fungi, bacteria, allergies, or viruses, among other things. Diseases of the epidermis can alter the texture and color of the skin. In general, skin diseases are chronic, contagious, and can occasionally progress to skin malignancy [1]. The human body contains numerous organs, including the brain, muscles, neurons, tissues, lungs, and so on. The epidermis, the human body's largest organ, is also a vital component that protects the inner organs.

Fungi, invisible bacteria, allergic reactions, skin-texture-altering microbes, and pigment-producing microbes can cause skin diseases. Skin problems may be detected in the early stages. Most individuals are ignorant of the type and stage of a skin disease. A portion of skin diseases may manifest symptoms months after the initial infection, allowing the disease to develop and spread. This is due to the dearth of medical awareness among the general population. A skin disease is challenging to diagnose and may necessitate expensive laboratory testing to establish the type and stage of the condition.

A. Souri and S. Bendak (Eds.): IoTHIC 2023, ECPSCI 8, pp. 28–38, 2024.
https://doi.org/10.1007/978-3-031-52787-6_3

The development of laser and photonics-based medical technologies has made skin disease diagnosis considerably quicker and more accurate. However, the current expense of such a diagnosis is prohibitively expensive. Alternatively, we offer a method based on image processing for diagnosing skin diseases. This technique employs image analysis to identify the type of disease by analyzing a digital photograph of the diseased skin. Indeed, the expense of a comprehensive diagnosis is limited and prohibitively expensive at present. AI-based techniques help with image processing-based skin disease diagnosis. This technique employs image analysis to identify the type of disease by analyzing a digital photograph of the diseased skin. AI-based methods are efficient, fast, and accurate and require only a digital camera and a computer as expensive equipment [2].

In recent years, convolutional neural networks (CNN) have become widely used in a variety of feature extraction and classification applications. CNN extracts tiny information from images using convolution kernels of varying sizes, including the capacity to distinguish finger veins. For vein recognition, CNNs were known to have complex topologies [3]. Artificial neural networks can solve problems involving pattern recognition, classification, clustering, dimensionality reduction, computer vision, natural language processing (NLP), regression, and predictive analysis [4].

Another study contributed to Medicare used a Vgg19 deep neural network and light (GBM) to create a hybrid algorithm. Algorithm for the classification of brain tumors. They ran two types of tests, with the first trial dividing the MRI scans into tumor and normal categories, with a 100% success rate. As for the second experiment, the tumors were classified into four groups, with a success rate of 97.33%. A data set of 7023 MRI images was used [5].

The actual research aims to study the classification of up to 7 different skin diseases, namely basal cell carcinoma BCC, dermatofibroma DF, melanoma MN, pigmented benign keratosis PBK, seborrheic keratosis SK, squamous cell carcinoma SCC and vascular VU lesion. The use of a CNN deep neural network with variable output layer size allows to customize the number of detected classes. The paper shows that the binary classification achieves the highest accuracy of 99% which decays progressively to a value near 87% for the 7 classes in the dataset.

This paper is organized as follows: the first section is an introduction, while the second section presents previous literature study of similar research. In the third section, a presentation of the methodology is explained together with the proposed CNN architecture. The 4th section shows the simulation results concerning the loss and the accuracy of the proposed solution in different cases, and the 5th section discusses the findings of this research. Finally, Sect. 6 presents the conclusion.

2 Related Works

The method in [6] addressed the issue of classifying skin lesions into eight groups, Melanoma, nevi, basal cell carcinoma, squamous cell carcinoma, actinic keratosis, benign keratosis, dermatofibroma, and vascular lesions are all skin cancers. The ISIC-2019 data set was utilized. Also, additional samples images were used. Authors established an ensemble of CNN architectures. Six Efficient Net configurations, two Resent, and a SENet made up the ideal ensemble. Using five-fold cross-validation, they were able to reach an accuracy of 75.2%. The system won first place in the ISIC 2019 Skin Lesion Classification Challenge with an overall accuracy of 63.6% on task 1 and 63.4% on task on the official test set.

In [7, 8], federated learning is used to improve the performance and keeping security of diagnosis. In [7] CNN-based skin disease classification paired with the federated learning approach is a technique to classify skin diseases in humans while protecting personal information. The study has proposed a model for acne, eczema, and psoriasis classification. Its applying a technique of image augmentation allowed an accuracy of 86%, 43%, and 60%, as well as a recall of 67%, 60%, and 60%, respectively for the three mentioned classes. The model in the federated learning strategy had an average accuracy of 81.21%, 86.57%, 91.15%, and 94.15% when the dataset was distributed among 1000, 1500, 2000, and 2500 patients.

Authors of [9] suggested for the classification of skin lesions, an ensemble made up of enhanced CNNs and a regularly spaced test-time-shifting approach. It uses a shift technique to create several test input images, feeds them for each classifier in the ensemble, and then aggregates all the classifiers' outputs to vote on the class of the disease. On the HAM10000 dataset, it had a classification accuracy of 83.6%.

Karthik et al. [10], to classify the disease, suggested CNN with approximately 16 M parameters, which is significantly fewer than existing deep learning algorithms described in their state-of-the-art. The four groups utilized to categorize skin illnesses in this research were actinic keratosis (AK), acne, melanoma, and psoriasis. The overall accuracy of the model during testing was 84.70%.

Hameed et al. [11] described a method by using computer-aided diagnosis (CAD), Acne, eczema, psoriasis, benign and malignant melanoma, as well as eczema and psoriasis, were reported to be diagnosed by the system. The region of interest from which features are collected and extracted utilizing Otsu's threshold strategy, after application of the Dull Razor algorithm and the Gaussian filtering in the preprocessing to eliminate the trace of hairs from images. Several color and texture features were taken out and fed into the quadratic kernel of the Support Vector Machine (SVM). The experiment included 1800 photos, and the six-class categorization had an accuracy rate of 83%. However, the system was constrained by the dataset's small size.

The study presented in [12] has shown efficiency in classifying seven different types of skin conditions. Color features as well as texture features are extracted from the training images. A huge dataset can increase with the appropriate advanced computing procedures to deliver improved accuracy, CNN's accuracy achieved 84%. This approach aids in the accurate comparison of skin disease images, improving the standards for quality in the medical and research fields.

Sarker et al. [13] used transformers based neural networks to extract interesting features from images. The transformers-based model uses bidirectional encoder representation from the dermatoscopic image to perform the classification task. Experiments using the public dataset HAM10000, brought up results of 90.22%, 99.54%, 94.05%, and 96.28% in accuracy, precision, recall, and F1 score respectively, were achieved.

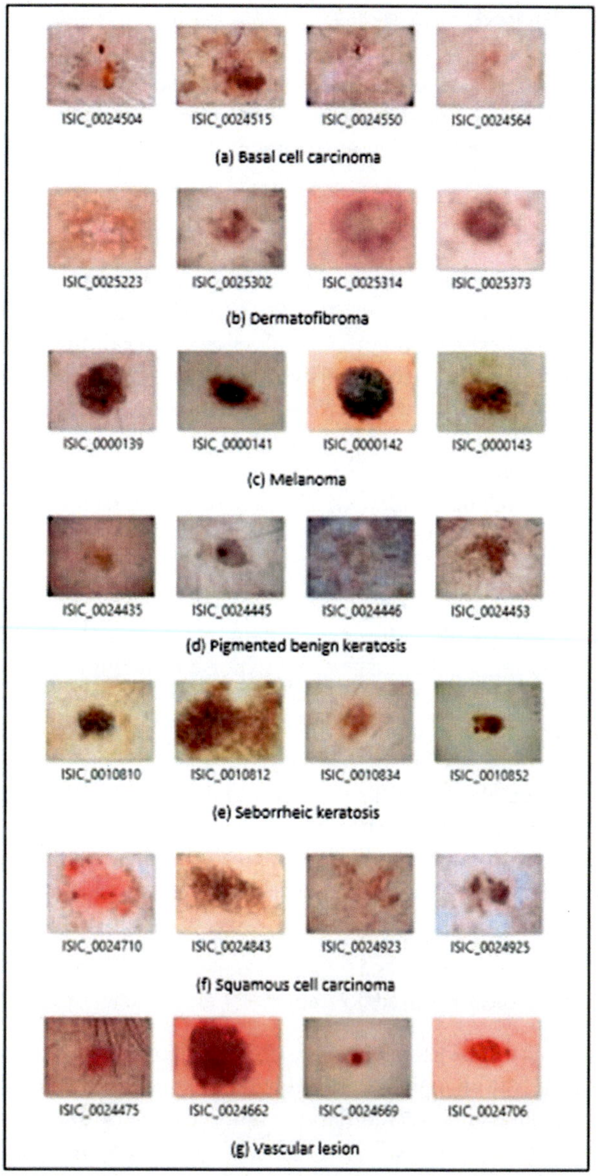

Fig. 1. Samples of the dataset representing the skin diseases classes [4].

Yanagisawa et al. [14] uses a CNN segmentation model to generate skin diseases images with specific requirements and used the obtained dataset to classify diseases by CAD algorithm and showed that the CNN segmentation model performs as well as hand-cropped images. This research used the dataset NSDD organized by the Japanese dermatological association.

3 Proposed Method

The proposed system focuses on proposing a disease classification model with high percentage of accuracy. The model is constructed using the CNN algorithm, it should be capable of achieving high prediction accuracy.

3.1 Dataset Description

In this section, the datasets used to train and test the accuracy of the proposed system will be described. The cutaneous diseases dataset namely (ISIC 2019) includes 2357 images organized into seven categories. Figure 1 displays examples of the dataset's categories. This dataset was obtained from the website (https://www.kaggle.com/datasets/bhanuprasanna/isic-2019), it was divided into two parts: a training part and a testing part.

Training Part: 80% of the dataset, or 1872 images, were used to train the CNN algorithm using this section.

Testing Part: 20% of the dataset, or 234 images, were used in this section for the purpose of training the CNN algorithm.

3.2 Image Processing

A preliminary processing of the image implies noise cancelling, the noise is removed from the images using three varieties of filters (Mean, Median, and Gaussian). The purpose of noise removal is to improve the accuracy of feature extraction from images and prevent noise from affecting the extracted features. In the segmentation step we used the Otsu's segmentation algorithm. Also, all images within the dataset, due to their varying sizes, will be resized to a specific dimension (64×64). Pixels of the images will be normalized by dividing the pixel's intensity by 255 to obtain features' values sweeping between 0 and 1 in order to shorten the training phase and to decrease the memory requirements.

3.3 Architecture of the Proposed System

This section presents the suggested model for improving skin disease classification accuracy using deep learning applied to a convolutional neural network. The proposed model consists of eight main layers: three convolutional layers, three pooling layers, and two fully connected layers. Figure 2 shows the architecture of the CNN model.

In the proposed system, three convolution layers were utilized to extract the required features from images. To construct a feature map, three layers with different kernel sizes were created: the first layer has a kernel size of 256, the second layer has a kernel size of 128 and the size of the third convolutional layer's kernel is 64.

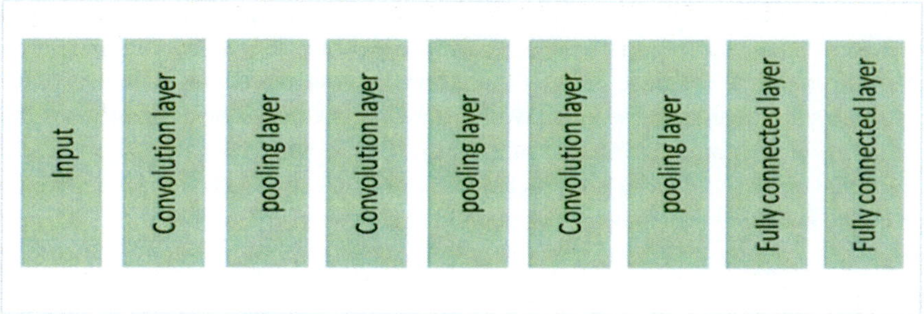

Fig. 2. Proposed Convolutional Neural Networks Model.

Only significant and dominant features are selected by the pooling layer, and three levels of pooling are used to determine which features have the greatest impact on vein class determination.

A dropout layer serves as an auxiliary layer after the pooling layer by eliminating features with little effect on classification precision and vein class prediction. The first through third dropout layers now have three extra dropout layers with dropout probability of 0.025, 0.4, and 0.5, respectively, as shown in Table 1.

Table 1. Convolution layers characteristics.

Layer		Function of Activation	Kernel Size	Probability	Parameters matrix
Convolution	First	Relu	128		
	Second Convolution	Relu	64		
	Third Convolution	Relu	32		
Pooling	First	Max	5 × 5		
	Second Pool	Max	2 × 2		
	Third Pool	Max	2 × 2		
Dropout	First			0.45	
	Second			0.8	
	Third			0.8	
Fully connected	First	Relu	128		
	Second	Softmax	7		903

The system then applies the flatten operation to the output of the preceding Neural Network to change the features from a 2D array to a 1D array. Two layers in the proposed system are completely connected. Relu and SoftMax, respectively, serve as the activation mechanisms for the first and second layers. The structure of the chosen solution is shown in Table 1 along with details about each layer.

Samples from the dataset are processed through successive layers, and a weight is assigned to each disease category based on the derived image attributes.

4 Experimental Results

The practical experiments of training the deep learning CNN algorithm will be detailed in this section, where the algorithm was taught by varying the number of training classes, as follows:

- Case1: the proposed system is trained using two classes namely (basal cell carcinoma dermatofibroma). The second fully connected layer provides predictions of the two classes only. The Loss evolution and the accuracy evolution in function of epoch number are represented in Table 2.
- Case2: the proposed system is trained using three classes namely (basal cell carcinoma, dermatofibroma, and melanoma).
- Case3: the proposed system learns using four classes namely (basal cell carcinoma, dermatofibroma, and Melanoma and Pigmented benign keratosis).
- Case4: the proposed system acquires knowledge from five classes namely (basal cell carcinoma, dermatofibroma, melanoma, pigmented benign keratosis and seborrheic keratosis).
- Case 5: the proposed system is trained using six classes namely (basal cell carcinoma, dermatofibroma, melanoma, pigmented benign keratosis, seborrheic keratosis and squamous cell carcinoma).
- Case6: the proposed system learns from samples of seven classes namely (basal cell carcinoma, dermatofibroma, melanoma, pigmented benign keratosis, seborrheic keratosis, squamous cell carcinoma and vascular lesion).

Results of cases 1 through 6 are shown in Table 2. The accuracies of training and testing tend to 1 progressively and at the same time the losses of training and testing converge towards 0. In particular for case 6 and at epoch 100, the accuracy reaches the limit of 85.69% on testing samples, which is the maximum accuracy of testing achieved by the suggested system. Table 3 illustrates a summary of the best results concerning training loss and accuracy, and testing loss and accuracy.

Table 2. Training – testing results of the different cases.

Number Of Class	ACC	Loss
2-class	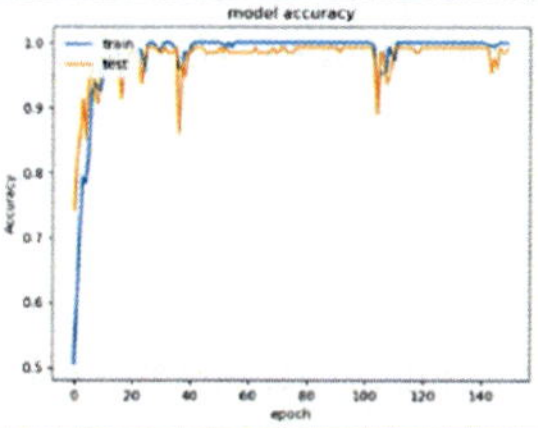	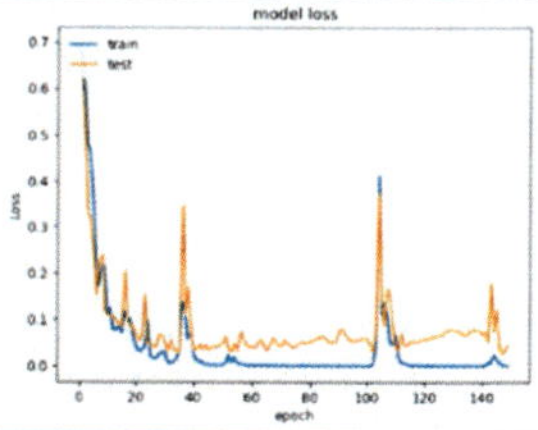
3-Class	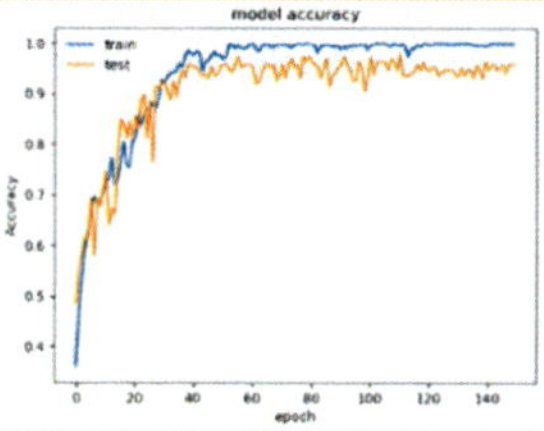	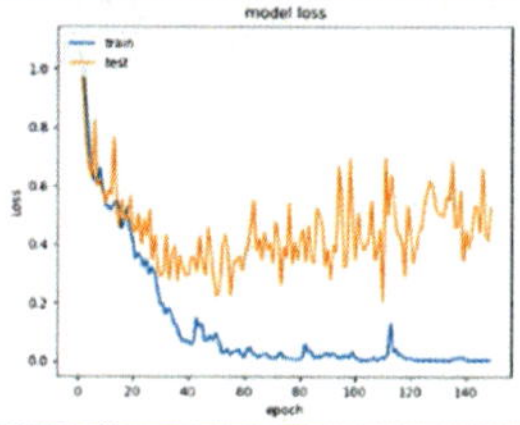
4-Class	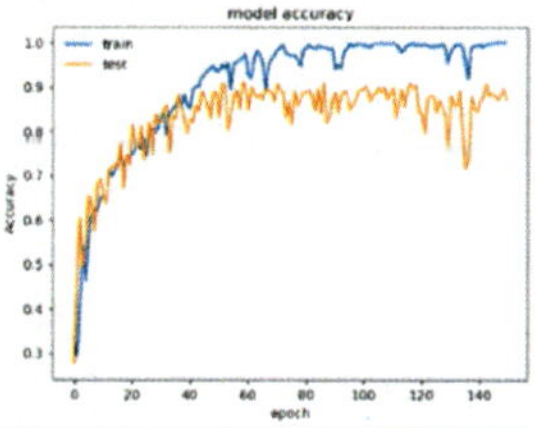	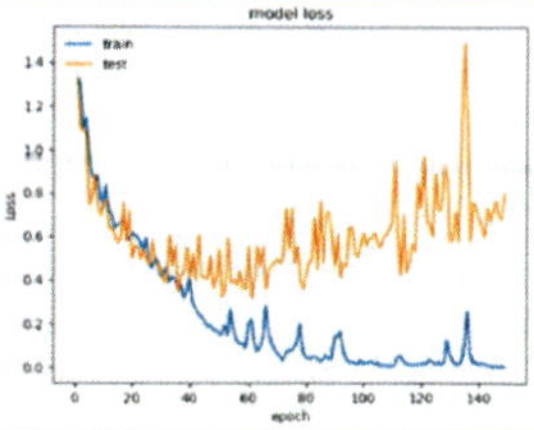
5-Class	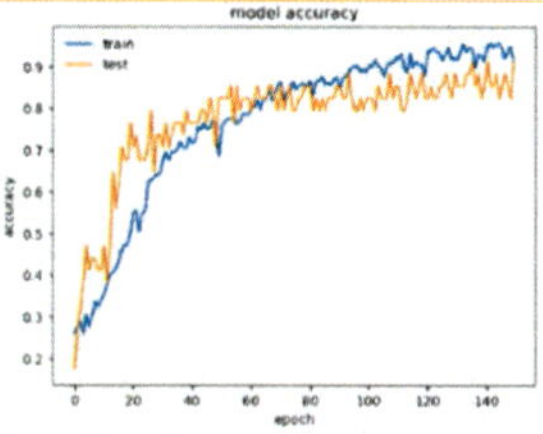	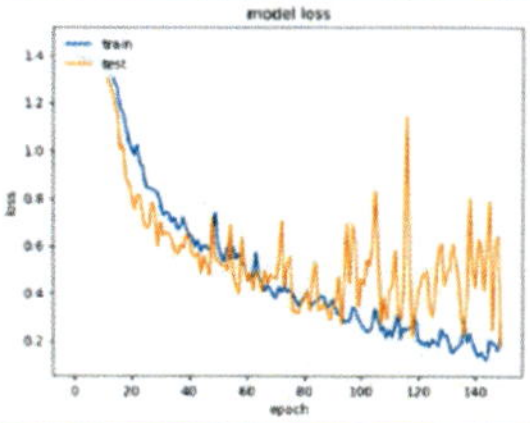
6-Class	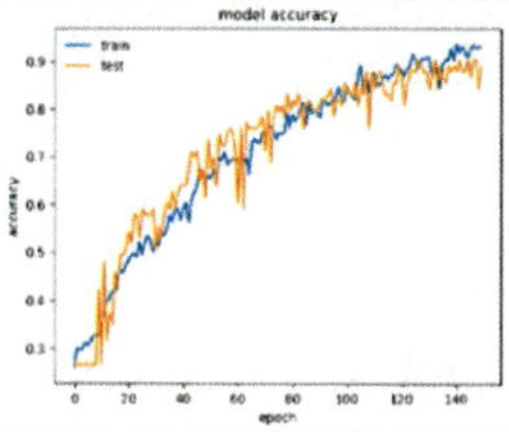	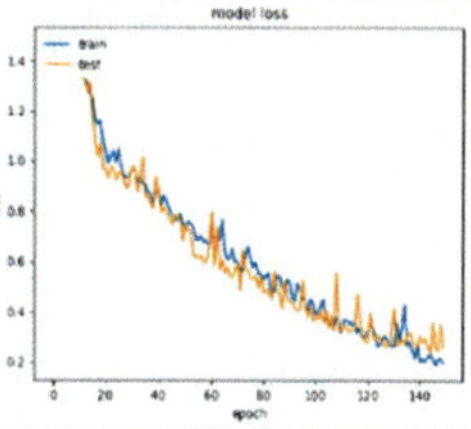
7-Class	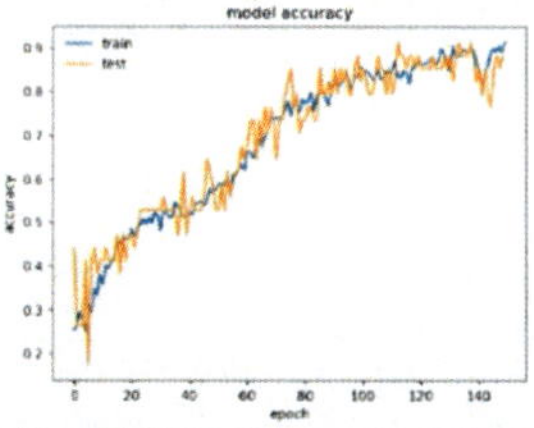	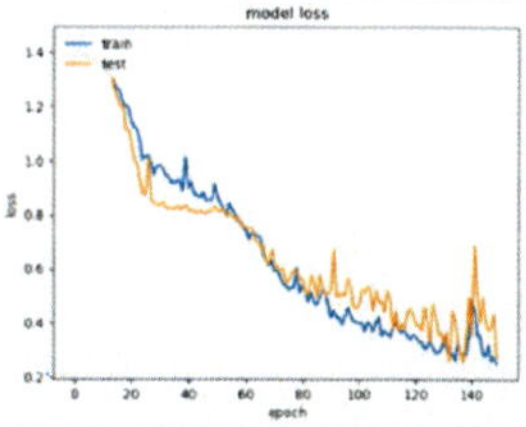

5 Result Discussion

In this section, the results of the proposed skin diseases classification are compared with previous works. For the purpose of comparison, the following published research papers have been selected [6–11]. In [6], the research used several preprocessing techniques to image enhancement and used modified CNN for diseases classification, while the research [7] used skin lesions, an ensemble made up of enhanced CNNs and a regularly spaced test-time-shifting approach. While research [10] used computer-aided diagnosis (CAD) system was reported by for diagnosing the most prevalent skin lesions. The research [9] and [11] used CNN model for classification. Table 4 illustrates comparison between results of proposed work with previous works. The achieved accuracy by the proposed CNN outperforms all the previous studies by at least 3.2%.

Table 3. Summary of Training-Test Results.

Case	Epoch	Training		Validation	
		Loss Rate	Accuracy	Loss rate	Accuracy
Case1	20	0.0596	0.9864	0.1519	0.9685
	60	0.0024	1.0000	0.1896	0.9764
	150	7.7416e-04	1.0000	0.0455	0.9921
Case2	20	0.4441	0.8203	0.4362	0.7796
	60	0.0232	0.9885	0.0590	0.9677
	150	8.2215e-04	1.0000	0.5275	0.9570
Case3	20	0.5379	0.7720	0.5819	0.7590
	60	0.1337	0.9620	0.4416	0.8514
	150	0.0046	1.0000	0.7960	0.8715
Case4	20	1.0940	0.4529	1.0080	0.6429
	60	0.5830	0.7705	0.5398	0.7831
	150	0.2363	0.9169	0.1792	0.9118
Case5	20	1.0242	0.5491	0.9646	0.4880
	60	0.5821	0.7610	0.5250	0.7600
	150	0.1939	0.9315	0.2572	0.8916
Case6	20	1.1673	0.4849	1.0882	0.5663
	60	0.8368	0.6329	0.8351	0.6184
	150	0.2519	0.9131	0.2712	0.8729

Table 4. Comparison with previous works.

Research	Algorithms	Accuracy
[6]	Ensemble of CNNs	75.2%
[7]	Federated CNN	Up to 94%
[9]	Ensemble of CNNs	83.60%
[10]	CNN	84.7%
[11]	SVM	83%
Proposed System	Proposed CNN model	**85.8%**

6 Conclusion

Through Sect. 4, we noticed the convergence in the accuracy of the results, which makes the proposed system able to recognize skin diseases precisely, as the accuracy rate of the proposed system in discrimination reached more than 87%. This accuracy is considered excellent and the proposed system using deep learning was successful in the classification of the diseases. Moreover, through the previous comparison, it was pointed out that the proposed system using the CNN deep learning algorithm reached a higher accuracy than state of the art. The performance of the proposed model can be explained by the fact that CNN deep learning algorithm contains a series of layers through which the system extracts the features of vein fingerprint images and select the best features, meanwhile, the fully connected layers apply to the classification of the disease.

References

1. Prasad, P.M.K., Jahnavi, S., Gayatri, N., Sravani, T.: Skin Disease Detection using Image Processing and Machine Learning (2023)
2. Almeida, M.A.M., Santos, I.A.X.: Classification models for skin tumor detection using texture analysis in medical images. J. Imaging **6**(6), 51 (2020)
3. Noh, K.J., Choi, J., Hong, J.S., Park, K.R.: Finger-vein recognition based on densely connected convolutional network using score-level fusion with shape and texture images. IEEE Access **8**, 96748–96766 (2020)
4. Shrestha, A., Mahmood, A.: Review of deep learning algorithms and architectures. IEEE Access **7**, 53040–53065 (2019)
5. Abdulkader, H., Hussein, A.: Brain Tumor Classification Using Hybrid Algorithms (VGG19) and Light (GBM) (2022). https://doi.org/10.14704/NQ.2022.20.11.NQ66655
6. Gessert, N., Nielsen, M., Shaikh, M., Werner, R., Schlaefer, A.: Skin lesion classification using ensembles of multi-resolution EfficientNets with meta data. MethodsX **7**, 100864 (2020)
7. Hossen, M.N., Panneerselvam, V., Koundal, D., Ahmed, K., Bui, F.M., Ibrahim, S.M.: Federated machine learning for detection of skin diseases and enhancement of internet of medical things (IoMT) security. IEEE J. Biomed. Health Inform. **27**(2), 835–841 (2023). https://doi.org/10.1109/JBHI.2022.3149288
8. Yaqoob, M.M., Alsulami, M., Khan, M.A., Alsadie, D., Saudagar, A.K.J., AlKhathami, M.: Federated machine learning for skin lesion diagnosis: an asynchronous and weighted approach. Diagnostics **13**(11), 1964 (2023). https://doi.org/10.3390/diagnostics13111964

9. Thurnhofer-Hemsi, K., López-Rubio, E., Domínguez, E., Elizondo, D.A.: Skin lesion classification by ensembles of deep convolutional networks and regularly spaced shifting. IEEE Access **9**, 112193–112205 (2021)
10. Karthik, R., Vaichole, T.S., Kulkarni, S.K., Yadav, O., Khan, F.: Eff2Net: an efficient channel attention-based convolutional neural network for skin disease classification. Biomed. Signal Process. Control **73**, 103406 (2022)
11. Hameed, N., Shabut, A., Hossain, M.A.: A computer-aided diagnosis system for classifying prominent skin lesions using machine learning. In: 2018 10th Computer Science and Electronic Engineering (CEEC), 2018, pp. 186–191 (2018)
12. Kalaiyarivu, M., Nalini, N.J.: Classification of skin disease image using texture and color features with machine learning techniques. Math. Stat. Eng. Appl., **71**(3s2), 682–699 (2022)
13. Sarker, M.M.K., Moreno-García, C.F., Ren, J., Elyan, E.: TransSLC: skin lesion classification in dermatoscopic images using transformers. In: Yang, G., Aviles-Rivero, A., Roberts, M., Schönlieb, C.-B. (eds.) Medical Image Understanding and Analysis: 26th Annual Conference, MIUA 2022, Cambridge, UK, July 27–29, 2022, Proceedings, pp. 651–660. Springer, Cham (2022). https://doi.org/10.1007/978-3-031-12053-4_48
14. Yanagisawa, Y., Shido, K., Kojima, K., Yamasaki, K.: Convolutional neural network-based skin image segmentation model to improve classification of skin diseases in conventional and non-standardized picture images. J. Dermatol. Sci. **109**(1), 30–36 (2023)

Using Explainable Artificial Intelligence and Knowledge Graph to Explain Sentiment Analysis of COVID-19 Post on the Twitter

Yi-Wei Lai[1(✉)] and Mu-Yen Chen[2]

[1] Department of Engineering Science, National Cheng Kung University, Tainan, Taiwan
N98101054@gs.ncku.edu.tw

[2] Department of Engineering Science, National Cheng Kung University, Tainan, Taiwan
mychen119@gs.ncku.edu.tw

Abstract. Social media has become the common way for people to share information and opinions. For analyze opinions about events or products, sentiment analysis has become a hot topic. The existing methods mainly use deep learning models to directly analyze the data collected on the social media and get results. However, deep learning models are generally "black boxes", and it is impossible to know the relationship between data and results and the adjustment of internal parameters of the model. Therefore, the concept of explainable AI has become important. Explain the results of deep learning models through explainable AI models. In addition, knowledge graphs are constructed through reliable external databases. A reliable relationship diagram can also provide a good explanation effect. The study uses explainable AI and knowledge graphs to assist in explaining the application of deep learning models in sentiment analysis to understand which features in the data are important features, as well as the influence and attributes of these features. In the results, explainable AI specifically shows the impact of each feature in the sentence on the result, and the knowledge graph uses the sentiment of keywords, the sentiment of the post itself and the Subject–Verb–Object knowledge graph formed by the common verbs in the post to assist in explaining the results of the deep learning model. Finally, the concept of explainable AI and knowledge graph can help users better understand how features affect model detection.

Keywords: Sentiment analysis · Explainable AI · Knowledge graph · Social media

1 Introduction

With the development of communication technology and the popularization of mobile devices, social media such as Facebook, Twitter, Instagram has become common in people's lives. According to statistics, there are 4.8 billion social media users in the world [1], and the average daily use time of social media per person is 2 h and 31 min in 2023 [2]. It shows that people have become accustomed to these technological applications.

A. Souri and S. Bendak (Eds.): IoTHIC 2023, ECPSCI 8, pp. 39–49, 2024.
https://doi.org/10.1007/978-3-031-52787-6_4

Nowadays, many people will express their opinions and thoughts on events or products, and the anonymity and convenience of social media will further enhance the willingness of the public to express and COVID-19 has become a major public health event, so it has also provided a lot of research on prevention and damage reduction, whether it is through actual CT images for predicting whether to be infected [3] or using machine learning to detect COVID-19 outbreaks [4], and use epidemic-related data to conduct relevant analysis [5]. so, in the field of text analysis, many studies will use the posts on these social medias to conduct sentiment analysis, public opinion analysis, used to analyze public impressions and thoughts on related events or products. Many studies use deep learning models for analysis to obtain more accurate results, but deep learning models are called black box, and the results will be obtained directly after the data enters the model. The result is a predicted probability value, but it is impossible to know any causal relationship between the data and the result, and it is difficult to know which key features specifically affect it, which is critical for analysis, so the concept of explainable AI (XAI) was proposed. Through XAI, the deep learning model is deconstructed to understand how the model detect the result based on the data, in addition to XAI, the knowledge graph also has a similar effect. By deconstructing the Subject–Verb–Object (SVO) of the data, it can be seen how the features in the data are connected and the relationship is calculated to achieve explainable.

Therefore, this study uses deep learning to analyze health-related issues and the recent popular event COVID-19 on multiple social platforms, to understand the posts that the public follows on social platforms and their own emotions, and then through XAI With detailed analysis of the knowledge graph, by explaining how features affect the results and utilizing external knowledge bases to construct SVO and sentiment relationships of posts, it can be understood what people pay more attention to in social media posts under a certain topic.

The contributions of this study are as follows:

- The research compares different explainable AI models and shows how different models explain detection results from deep learning models.
- The research used the knowledge graph to analyze the common SVO and sentiment relationship of posts.

The structure of the research is as follows. Section 2 discusses related literature. Section 3 describes the specific research framework, including the data preprocessing, the research model, explainable AI model and the Knowledge graph. Section 4 shows the experiment results. Section 5 describes the conclusions.

2 Literature Review

2.1 Sentiment Analysis

The social media enables users to discuss and share opinions on various issues at any time, whether it is product reviews or social events, there are all kinds of tweets on social media, and users will express their opinions on various topics, so many studies will collect and analyze the data on social media, and the most common analysis is sentiment analysis by classifying the words and sentences in the community posts to understand the sentiment of the posts, and by analyzing the sentiment of a large number of posts, we can know the public's overall views on related issues, which can be extended into public opinion analysis.

There have been many research on sentiment analysis [6, 7], In addition to politics, health-related issues are also the main areas that are often analyzed, Wankhade et al. conducted a comprehensive discussion on various aspects of sentiment analysis, including the categories of sentiment analysis, data selection and feature extraction of sentiment analysis, method selection of sentiment analysis, evaluation indicators and application fields of sentiment analysis, in the analysis, each project is introduced in detail, its advantages and disadvantages are analyzed, as well as opportunities and challenges, and the conclusions also give researchers a clear direction for development [8]. Bordoloi & Biswas conducted an overall assessment of sentiment analysis papers in recent years, discussed each methodology in detail, and made critical comments on the design framework of sentiment analysis and lists the characteristic variables and challenges that have not yet been fully broken through in sentiment analysis, and extends to possible future research and application fields [9].

2.2 Explainable AI

Explainable AI is a novel technology that is often mentioned in recent years. Since most of the past deep learning models are so-called black boxes, The result is generated directly after the input data, and it is not known how the data affects the result and how the internal parameters of the model work. Therefore, the concept of explainable AI was proposed. The common explainable AI, such as LIME, Shapley, etc., whether it is in computer vision, natural language processing, and other topics have good explanatory effect.

Çılgın et al. use the Valence-Aware Dictionary Emotional Reasoner (VADER) to conduct sentiment analysis on COVID-19 community posts. By using VADER's thesaurus design, they can understand the emotional meaning of each word in the post in detail, and it is not simply classified as positive and negative, but uses more diverse 5 classifications for sentiment analysis [10]. The Locally Explainable Model-Agnostic Explanation (LIME) model is used to explain the classification of deep learning models through local explainable [11]. However, as the amount of data increases, the effect of LIME will vary greatly due to different sampling, therefore, Shi et al. proposed a new extension of LIME to enhance the explainable and fidelity of the model by combining LIME's local interpretation sampling and nonlinear approximation (LEDSNA) [12]. The transformer deep learning model provides good results in detection in many fields, but like other deep learning models, it does not have the interpretation of the relationship between data and results, but the existing explanatory AI models all focus on word features or take the way of external analysis, which is less directly combined with the transformer deep learning model. Therefore, a novel explainable AI model is proposed. The model adapts the explainable AI model Shapley [13] to the transformer-based deep learning model enables the model to simultaneously perform explainable calculations during detection and improves the problem that other models cannot provide better explanations based on the text context [14].

2.3 Knowledge Graph

A lot of data in the real world is unorganized messy information. The concept of knowledge graph is to analyze the data through the relationship diagram, sort out the relationship between the data in an effective way, and obtain meaningful information. In terms of natural language processing, because the language has the characteristics of SVO, it is possible to associate different subjects during parsing, find out the relationship between different entities, and construct these relationships into a network architecture. Through these large networks, it is possible to clearly define which feature forms and relationships entities will have in most cases and can reduce false detections that may be caused by deep learning models.

Sentiment analysis methods often use machine learning or deep learning models for analysis, but these models cannot fully analyze the richness of the text, and can only identify them individually based on the character features of the text, therefore, the relationship network of the knowledge graph can be imported into the model to form a hybrid model. By combining the image similarity with the detection results of the deep learning model, make the results accurate and explainable. Weinzierl and Harabagiu constructed a misinformation detection model based on a knowledge graph, which detects attitudes between users through the knowledge graph, and the detection results based on the agreement and disagreement relationship between user attitudes and the results of the deep learning model used to detect COVID-19 information. The results show that the accuracy has reached a better level [15]. Hu et al. constructed a model based on knowledge graph and topic modeling model to detect fake news. First, the topic of the news was classified using topic modeling to identify real and fake news in advance. Then use the knowledge graph to build a relationship diagram. The relationship diagram is mainly to analyze the SVO in the sentence to establish a reliable interactive network structure. The entity structure established by real news and fake news will be different. Finally, the results of the two methods are combined to effectively improve the accuracy of detection [16]. Sentiment analysis using convolutional neural network (CNN) is also an effective method, but most of the research focuses on the features in the sentence and does not use external databases such as those used to build Knowledge graphs, resulting in if there are word skipping grammar interception or too many features that do not appear when building the model, the model analysis will be incorrect. Therefore, Gu et al. use the concept of knowledge graph to refer to external knowledge to build an emotional matrix to highlight important emotional word weights and use the word-sentence interaction network (WSIN) to calculate additional label features. The results show that the model has achieved excellent performance in sentiment analysis [17].

3 Methodology

3.1 Research Architecture

The method used in this study is to use a deep learning model to conduct sentiment analysis on community posts and combine Explainable AI and knowledge graphs to explain. This research will apply the model to social posts related to the health field obtained by the crawler and conduct sentiment analysis, in addition to the label results of sentiment analysis, the results will also use explainable AI models such as Shapley and LIME to explain part of speech and use knowledge graphs to analyze SVO features to achieve the effect of auxiliary explanation. Figure 1 shows the research architecture.

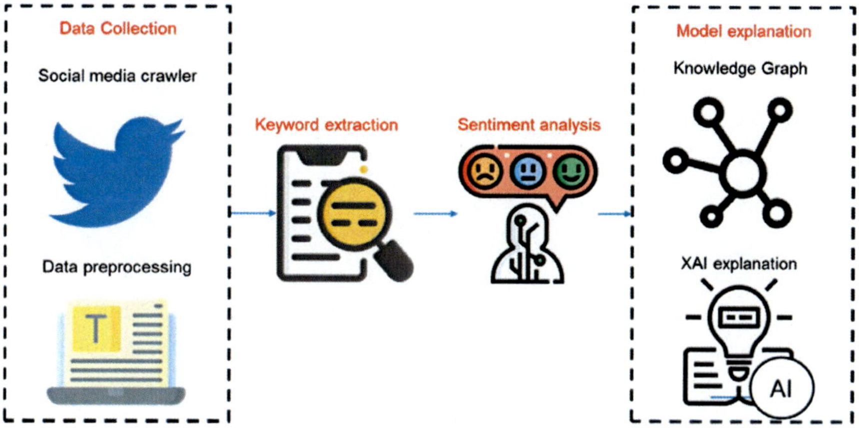

Fig. 1. The research architecture

3.2 Data Collection

In data collection, the study used a web crawler to locate posts related to COVID-19 on Twitter social media. The data collection time is from 2023-01-01 to 2023-06-30. By entering keywords into the search criteria, the crawler method will collect eligible posts and their author-related information. In the data preprocessing, since many posts will contain non-pure text such as hashtags and emoticons, they will be sorted to ensure that only text features are retained during analysis.

3.3 Keyword Extraction

Since the keywords in each post are not the same, and there are many miscellaneous items in the post, such as emoticons, hashtag and other factors, therefore, before performing keyword extraction, the post must be converted into plain text, that is, the above factors are removed, and then through the VADER thesaurus [18], the complete SVO in each post is defined through the thesaurus, and then according to SVO, the important words are extracted one by one to form a large number of keywords.

3.4 Sentiment Analysis

In terms of sentiment analysis, the Transformer-based deep learning model is a very powerful model. By inputting data in various fields into the Transformer model for training, the Transformer model uses a self-attention mechanism which can independently learn important features in each field data and generate different weights. Finally, a model that can be better used to detect different tasks in various fields is generated. Common models applied to natural language processing such as Bidirectional Encoder Representations from Transformers (BERT) [19], Robustly optimized BERT approach (RoBERTa), or various related extension models applied in different fields. The BERT architecture shows as Fig. 2. The research focuses on sentiment analysis to detect COVID-19-related posts, so the sentiment analysis model pre-trained by covid-19 posts is selected as the main model [20].

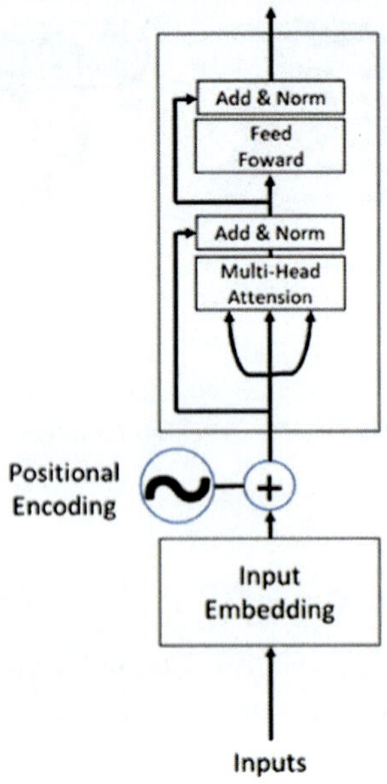

Fig. 2. The BERT architecture [19]

3.5 Explainable AI

The purpose of explainable artificial intelligence is to explain the effect of deep learning model detection in a way that humans can understand. Therefore, it will focus on explaining the results of deep learning using the characteristics of the data itself. In the language model, it will mainly consider the part of speech of word features, the relationship between categories and words, but the most important point of explainable AI is readability, so the explanation will be explained in a short and direct form.

LIME is an explainable model that uses locality analysis methods to parse the detection results of deep learning models. For example, deep learning will use non-intuitive representation features (such as word embedding). The model uses explainable representations (words) to explain these classifier results. In order to determine which features are important for prediction when explaining, the model will first scramble the sentences or reorganize the word order and assign weights to let the model predicts these sentences, and because many kinds of similar data are considered, it can be reasonably explained for individual important features when explaining [11].

LIME can be defined by the following Eq. 1. Since it uses local interpretation, the interpretation results of the model may not necessarily conform to the possible situation of the feature in the global state, but it will be more accurate in explaining the feature.

$$\xi(x) = argmin_{g \in G}\mathcal{L}\left(f, g, \prod_{x}\right) + \Omega(g) \quad (1)$$

The Eq. 1 assumes that the explainable AI model must consider the complexity of the data range, the similarity between the object of interpretation and its nearby instances, and minimize the degree of distortion when explaining, so as to make the explanation readable.

Another explainable AI model is based on the concept of game theory. Since each feature in the data has its own probability for different categories in sentence detection, therefore, the maximum value of each probability of the feature will be used to determine the contribution of the feature to the result. Shapley is this type of explainable AI model [13].

Shapley can explain the deep learning model through the following Eq. 2, which calculates the global features in calculations, and evaluates all features for why the deep learning model produces such results, and explain why the deep learning model will produce corresponding results. The lower the calculation result value of the feature, the negative correlation between the feature and the predicted target, and the higher the result value, the positive correlation between the feature and the predicted target.

$$\emptyset_i(f, x) = \sum_{z' \subseteq x^i} \frac{|z'|!(M - |z'| - 1)!}{M!}\left[f_x(z') - f_x(z' \backslash i)\right] \quad (2)$$

3.6 Knowledge Graph

The knowledge graph is constructed through the knowledge base, which stores a large amount of relevant resource data, and organizes these resources to present them in a graph relational structure, and the data is expressed in the form of SVO triples to form a semantic network. When constructing a knowledge graph, knowledge extraction is first performed, and a preliminary knowledge representation is formed by analyzing and integrating variables such as entities, relationships, and attributes in the data, and then disambiguating entities and aligning entities with complete pronouns and abbreviated sentences complete the standard knowledge representation. Then through knowledge reasoning and knowledge discovery, the data is evaluated and stored, and finally a large number of interrelated knowledge graphs are constructed based on the above results. From these knowledge graphs, the relationship between various entities can be understood, including sentiments, positions or actual relationships that exist between entities, etc.

4 Experiment Results

In the part of the experiment results, first, in the part of the crawler, after searching through keywords, the posts matching the keywords and their related information, such as author, time, number of reposts, number of likes, etc., will be used to generate results through sentiment analysis using a deep learning model and keyword extraction to extract important words.

Then, to assist identification, two XAI methods (Shapley, LIME) and knowledge graphs are used. In the Shapley explanation, each feature is automatically classified on both sides of the graph according to its influence, and the value will change in color according to the importance of the feature, so that users can better understand how the feature affects the result. The Shapley explanation is shown in Fig. 3. In the LIME explanation, the important features are mainly listed and sorted one by one according to the importance, and different colors are used to indicate the variables that affect the model detection. The LIME explanation diagram is shown in Fig. 4. Whether in LIME or Shapley, features will be displayed according to their influence, and the key features will be strengthened to highlight the most relevant features and their influence corresponding to the current issue, to understand what the most interesting content in these posts.

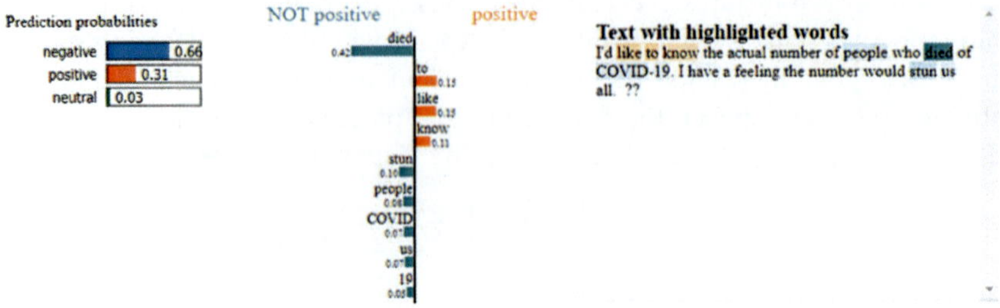

Fig. 3. The explainable result of the explainable AI LIME model

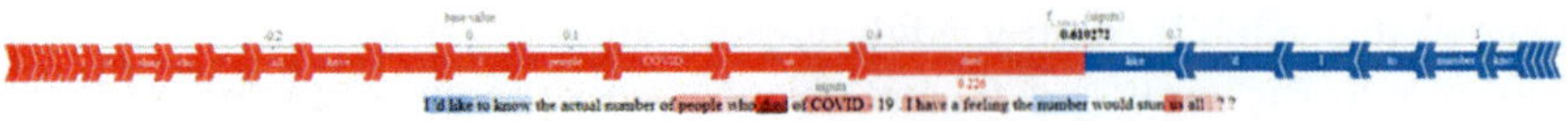

Fig. 4. The explainable result of the explainable AI Shapley model

Finally, on the knowledge graph, three connection graphs are designed. The first is a connection graph between keywords, which is used in sentiment analysis to examine the sentiment properties between key features and to determine what key features are common across many posts. As shown in Fig. 5, the second is based on the knowledge graph. The SVO of each entity is used to define a clear relationship between entities and form a complex relationship network. As shown in Fig. 6, the last one is the feature sentiment connection of each post. As shown in Fig. 7.

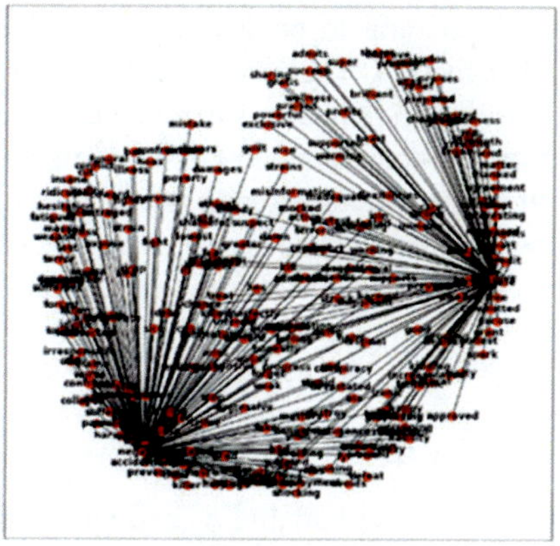

Fig. 5. The knowledge graph of the keyword sentiment analysis

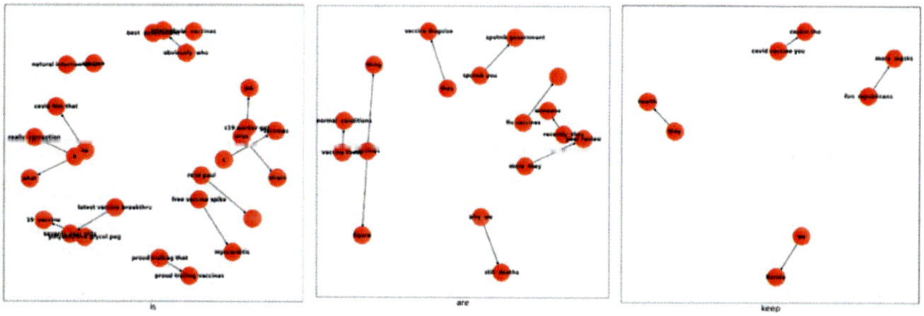

Fig. 6. The SVO knowledge graph of the post

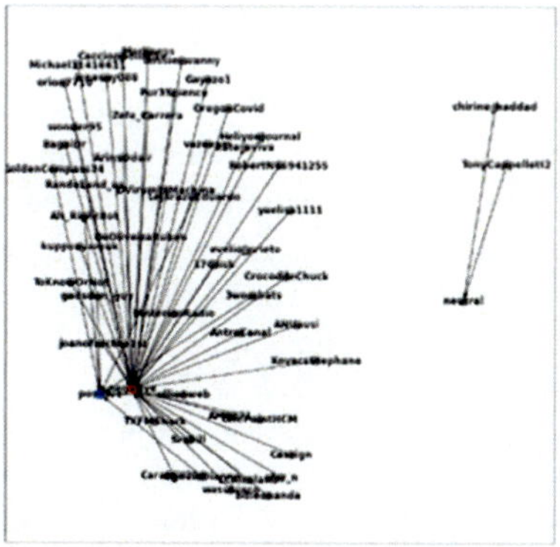

Fig. 7. The knowledge graph of the post sentiment analysis

It can be seen from the knowledge graph that in the part of post sentiment, since this study analyzes COVID-19, the sentiment of the information obtained from the crawler is mostly pessimistic. However, in terms of important features, most of the features can be seen there are corresponding to positive and negative directions respectively and have effect on model detection. Therefore, by classifying and sorting important features with clear emotions, emotion analysis can be better performed. As for the part of using the knowledge graph to construct SVO interaction, since the post will be short in performance, it may often only be expressed in one sentence. Therefore, the common verb, like is and are etc., will be selected as verbs to connect entities in construction. In this way, it is possible to analyze how the words in these posts are related to other words, and then understand what the focus of the issue is.

5 Conclusion

The research mainly explores how explainable AI and knowledge graph can assist deep learning in sentiment analysis and apply it to health-related community posts such as COVID-19. Since deep learning models often produce results after putting in data, it is impossible to know which features are more important. Therefore, through explainable AI, the attributes and influence of important features are displayed, and knowledge graphs are used to fully understand the interaction between features and the causal relationship between features and results, and finally help users understand why the results of sentiment analysis are corresponding labels.

In explaining the deep learning model, explainable AI will mainly explain all the features on a single data, and classify which features specifically affect the characteristic variables and influence of the positive and negative results of the model detection. On the knowledge graph, it mainly conducts a comprehensive analysis through all the data, defines a reliable benchmark through the external database, and uses this benchmark to analyze the data to strengthen the impact of interpretation features on the results. Therefore, it can be specifically understood in sentiment analysis on related issues, various postings focus on aspects and their emotions, so that subsequent larger-scale public opinion analysis can conduct in-depth analysis on the concerned aspects of related issues more accurately.

In future work, sentiment detection in multiple languages can be added to the data set. Since COVID-19 is a global event, there must be community posts in various languages discussing the event. By analyzing different languages, we can learn more about different views on COVID-19. Combining the knowledge graph with the deep learning model to create a new method that improves the error of the deep model when predicting with probability through a reliable external knowledge base.

Acknowledgement. This work was supported by the Ministry of Science and Technology, Taiwan, under Grant MOST110-2511-H-006-013-MY3 and MOST111-2622-H-006-004; and in part by the Higher Education Sprout Project, Ministry of Education to the Headquarters of University Advancement at National Cheng Kung University (NCKU).

References

1. Social Media. Statistics & Facts. Statista. https://www.statista.com/topics/1164/social-networks/#topicOverview. Accessed 24 July 2023

2. Digital 2022: Global Overview Report. DataReportal. https://datareportal.com/reports/digital-2022-global-overview-report. Accessed 24 July 2023
3. Heidari, A., Toumaj, S., Navimipour, N.J., Unal, M.: A privacy-aware method for COVID-19 detection in chest CT images using lightweight deep conventional neural network and blockchain. Comput. Biol. Med. **145**, 105461 (2022)
4. Heidari, A., Jafari Navimipour, N., Unal, M., Toumaj, S.: Machine learning applications for COVID-19 outbreak management. Neural Comput. Appl. **34**, 15313–15348 (2022)
5. Aminizadeh, S., et al.: The applications of machine learning techniques in medical data processing based on distributed computing and the Internet of Things. Comput. Methods Prog. Biomed. **241**, 107745 (2023)
6. Lai, Y., Chen, M.: Review of survey research in fuzzy approach for text mining. IEEE Access **11**, 39635–39649 (2023)
7. Xu, Q., Chang, V., Jayne, C.: A systematic review of social media-based sentiment analysis: emerging trends and challenges. Decis. Analyt. J. **3**, 100073 (2022)
8. Wankhade, M., Rao, A.C., Kulkarni, C.: A survey on sentiment analysis methods, applications, and challenges. Artif. Intell. Rev. **55**, 5731–5780 (2022)
9. Bordoloi, M., Biswas, S.K.: Sentiment analysis: a survey on design framework, applications and future scopes. Artif. Intell. Rev. 1–56 (2023)
10. Çilgin, C., Baş, M., Bilgehan, H., Ünal, C.: Twitter sentiment analysis during covid-19 outbreak with VADER. AJIT-e: Acad. J. Inf. Technol. **13**(49) (2022)
11. Ribeiro, M., Singh, S., Guestrin, C.: Why should i trust you?: Explaining the predictions of any classifier. In: The 22nd ACM SIGKDD International Conference on Knowledge Discovery and Data Mining, pp. 1135–1144. ACM, New York (2016)
12. Shi, S., Du, Y., Fan, W.: An extension of LIME with improvement of explainable and fidelity. arXiv preprint arXiv:2004.12277 (2020)
13. Lundberg, S.M., Lee, S.: A unified approach to interpreting model predictions. arXiv preprint arXiv:1705.07874 (2017)
14. Kokalj, E., Škrlj, B., Lavrač, N., Pollak, S., Robnik-Sikonja, M.: BERT meets Shapley: extending SHAPLEY explanations to transformer-based classifiers. In: The EACL Hackashop on News Media Content Analysis and Automated Report Generation, pp. 16–21. ACL, Online (2021)
15. Weinzierl, M.A., Harabagiu, S.M.: Identifying the adoption or rejection of misinformation targeting COVID-19 vaccines in twitter discourse. In: The ACM Web Conference 2022, pp.3196–3205. ACM, New York (2022)
16. Hu, L., et al.: Compare to the knowledge: graph neural fake news detection with external knowledge. In: Proceedings of the 59th Annual Meeting of the Association for Computational Linguistics and the 11th International Joint Conference on Natural Language Processing, pp. 754–763. ACL, Online (2021)
17. Gu, T., Zhao, H., He, Z., Li, M., Ying, D.: Integrating external knowledge into aspect-based sentiment analysis using graph neural network. Knowl.-Based Syst. **259**(10), 110025 (2022)
18. Hutto, C.J., Gilbert, E.: VADER: a parsimonious rule-based model for sentiment analysis of social media text. In: The International AAAI Conference on Web and Social Media, vol. 8, no. 1, pp. 216–225. AAAI, Michigan (2014)
19. Devlin, J., Chang, M., Lee, K., Toutanova, K.: BERT: pre-training of deep bidirectional transformers for language understanding. arxiv preprint arXiv:1810.04805 (2019)
20. Lamsal, R., Harwood, A., Read, M.R.: Twitter conversations predict the daily confirmed COVID-19 cases. Appl. Soft Comput. **129**, 109603 (2022)

Check for updates

An IoT-Based Telemedicine System for the Rural People of Bangladesh

Raqibul Hasan[1](✉), Md. Tamzidul Islam[2], and Md. Mubayer Rahman[2]

[1] Department of Software Engineering, Halic University, Istanbul, Turkey
raqibulhasn@halic.edu.tr

[2] Department of Computer Science and Engineering, Ahsanullah University of Science and Technology, Dhaka, Bangladesh
{180104123,180104144}@aust.edu

Abstract. IoT devices can enable low cost and interactive health care services. In this paper we have proposed an affordable telemedicine system to bring healthcare services within the reach of the rural people of Bangladesh. Proposed system enables transmission of patient's body parameters in real-time to a remote doctor. The proposed system also has real-time patient monitoring capability which is based on ECG signal classification. A feed-forward neural network is used for ECG signal classification on an embedded ARM processor. For low power operation, we have utilized fixed-point (integer) arithmetic instead of floating-point arithmetic for the ECG signal classification task. Proposed fixed-point implementation is 1.06x faster than floating-point implementation and requires 50% less memory to store the neural network model parameters without loss in the classification accuracy.

Keywords: IoT devices · telemedicine · ECG signal classification · remote patient monitoring · fixed-point operation

1 Introduction

Bangladesh is a developing country in the southeast Asia with about 160 million population. 60% of the total population lives in the rural area. Annual per capita income in the rural area is about $658 [1]. Developing countries like Bangladesh suffer from inadequate healthcare and medical services. Lack of healthcare professionals and infrastructure contribute to this problem making it more difficult to deliver healthcare to people in rural and remote communities. Particularly, there is a severe shortage of specialist doctors in the villages of Bangladesh [2, 3]. The doctors prefer to live in the cities because of better living, and better earnings.

Telemedicine is a rapidly growing field that has the potential to transform healthcare delivery. Wireless communication advancements and IoT devices have paved the path for more convenient and high-quality healthcare services [4, 5]. Telemedicine uses a variety of technologies, such as video conferencing, remote monitoring, and mobile health applications, to connect patients and healthcare providers across distances. This

A. Souri and S. Bendak (Eds.): IoTHIC 2023, ECPSCI 8, pp. 50–58, 2024.
https://doi.org/10.1007/978-3-031-52787-6_5

can be especially beneficial for patients who live in rural or remote areas, as it can provide access to healthcare services that would otherwise be difficult to obtain. Telemedicine can be used for a wide range of medical services, including consultation with specialist doctors, remote monitoring of chronic conditions, and mental health services. It can also be used to provide medical education and training to healthcare providers in remote areas. This technology also significantly lowers the cost of healthcare solutions. TytoCare is a remote patient examination device [6]. This device costs about $300 which is not affordable to many people living in the rural areas of Bangladesh.

Several research efforts identified the challenged of implementing a telemedicine solution in Bangladesh [7–9]. In the rural areas of Bangladesh, internet connectivity is not easily accessible. The rural people are not financially solvent enough to afford expensive telemedicine device like TytoCare. Most of the existing telemedicine solution in Bangladesh is limited to voice consultation over phone [7, 10]. Work in [11] described a telemedicine system for the rural people which requires a personal computer. This system lacks several important body sensors such as: heartbeat sensor, pulse rate sensor. Work in [12] analyzed the current situation and challenges of IoT based smart healthcare services for rural unprivileged people in Bangladesh. The authors only described the high-level idea using a very few sensors such as: pulse rate sensor. No detailed design or implementation was examined. In [13] a system has been proposed combining IoT, GSM, and mobile application. A real-time database was introduced which will provide information about the location of the patient, pharmacy, ambulance, and hospital. No body sensor was integrated into the system. In [14] an event-driven IoT architecture is presented for data analysis of reliable healthcare applications, including context, event, and service layers.

In this work, we used IoT devices and biomedical sensors to collect, analyze a patient's health data/parameters. These data are also transmitted to a remote doctor in real-time. The patient and doctor could be far away from each other. This telemedicine platform will bring health care benefits within the reach of the rural people where it is difficult to find a specialist doctor for consultation. It will alleviate the long travel of a patient from village to city where specialist doctors are usually located. Hence the proposed system will save people's time, energy, and healthcare cost. Single patient unit of the proposed system will cost about $50 which is significantly less compared to a TytoCare system [6].

The proposed system also has real-time patient monitoring capability. It is used for patient emergency situation detection [15]. The patient monitoring system is based on ECG (electrocardiogram) signal classification. We are classifying ECG signal on an embedded ARM processor in real-time. An embedded system has several constraints such as limited memory, slower clock frequency [16]. In a patient monitoring system, the embedded processor is battery powered. Hence an algorithm implemented on an embedded processor needs to be energy efficient. Work in [17] classifies ECG signal in real-time using deep learning algorithm on an embedded GPU. Embedded GPUs are more power consuming and expensive than an embedded ARM processor. Most of the existing ECG signal classification systems utilize floating-point operation [18].

Floating-point numbers provide more precision than integer numbers. But floating-point data storage requires more memory space than integer data. Furthermore, floating-point operations are slower and more energy consuming than integer operations [19]. Energy consuming operations will drain the battery quickly. In the proposed work, we implemented a feed-forward neural network (FNN) for ECG signal classification on an embedded ARM processor using integer (fixed-point) operations. This is another novel contribution of the proposed work.

The rest of the paper is organized as follows: Sect. 2 describes the proposed telemedicine system. Section 3 describes the real-time patient monitoring system. Section 4 describes the prototype design and presents the experimental result. Finally, in Sect. 5 we conclude our work.

2 Proposed Telemedicine System

In this work, we used IoT and biomedical sensors to collect, analyze, and transmit a patient's health data/parameters in real-time to a remote doctor. Body sensors collect a patient's vital signs, such as heart rate, blood pressure, and oxygen levels. These parameters allow healthcare providers to assess a patient's health and detect any changes or anomalies that may require intervention. Figure 1 shows the overall architecture of the proposed telemedicine system.

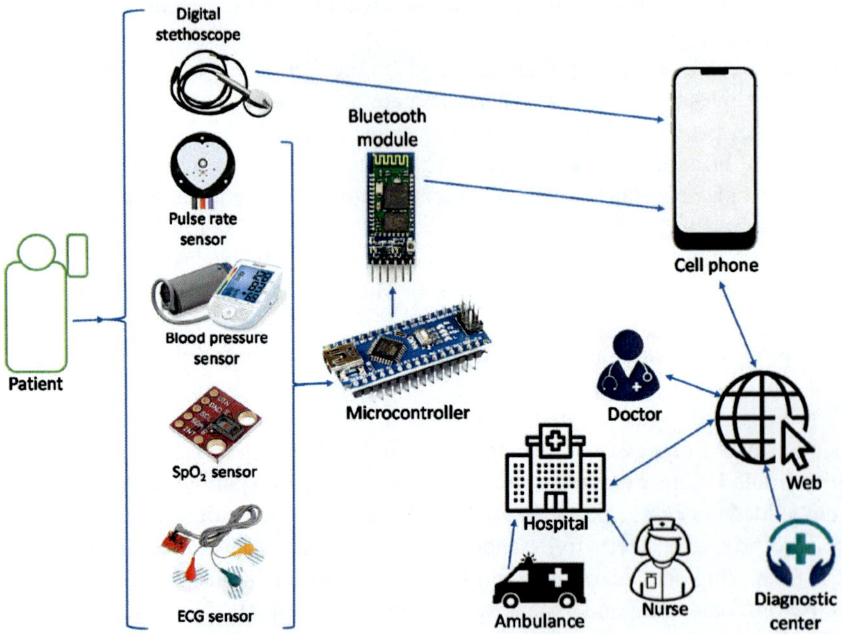

Fig. 1. Overall system diagram of the proposed telemedicine model.

A doctor heavily relies on a stethoscope signal for his/her initial examination of a patient. In the proposed system, a digital stethoscope is inserted directly into the cell phone's 3.5 mm headphone jack. The cell phone capture patient's heart and lung sound from the electric stethoscope and transmit the signal to the remote doctor's end in real-time. The system also has biomedical sensors such as pulse rate sensor, temperature sensor (LM35), SpO2 sensor for oxygen level measurement, blood pressure sensor and ECG sensor. These sensors are interfaced to a microcontroller. From the microcontroller these sensor data are transmitted to the cell phone using Bluetooth. The body sensor data are transmitted to the healthcare providers from the cell phone using the internet connectivity. The data are also displayed on the mobile screen through an app. A patient will be able to access his/her test report produced by a diagnostic center through the app. In the proposed system the patient, doctor, hospital, and diagnostic center are interconnected through the internet.

3 Real-Time Patient Monitoring

Patient monitoring is a very important feature in a healthcare system. It allows healthcare providers to monitor patients who have been discharged from the hospital or who are recovering from surgery. An IoT based remote patient monitoring system ensures that patients receive timely and appropriate care, regardless of their location or mobility. Furthermore, it can also be used for patient emergency situation detection [15].

The proposed system implements remote patient monitoring feature based on ECG signal classification. The real-time ECG signal classification system is battery powered. Hence, we need to use an embedded processor for the ECG signal classification task. Algorithm implementation on an embedded processor needs to be memory efficient as these systems have limited memory. Floating-point numbers provide more precision than integer numbers. But floating-point data storage requires more memory space than integer data. Furthermore, floating-point operations are slower and more energy consuming than integer operations [19]. In this work, we implemented a feed-forward neural network (FNN) for ECG signal classification on an embedded ARM processor using integer (fixed-point) operations.

Arrhythmia dataset [20] from UCI Machine Learning repository was used in this work to train the FNN. The dataset has total 452 instances (number of samples), 279 attributes each instance, and 16 classes (normal and 15 unusual classes). We used a FNN of configuration: 279->20->16 for the ECG signal classification task. The network has 20 neurons in the hidden layer and 16 neurons in the output layer. In the FNN the sigmoid activation function was used. Figure 2 shows the block diagram of the FNN. We used Keras Deep Learning tool [21] for training the FNN. Figure 3 shows the FNN training graph.

Figure 4 shows the methodology used in the proposed work for the implementation of the FNN on an ARM processor. For the fixed-point representation of the FNN weights, we considered 8 bits before the decimal point and 8 bits after the decimal point. Thus, one weight will require 2 bytes in this representation. The nonlinear sigmoid activation was implemented using a lookup table. The size of the lookup table is 512 byte (256 rows).

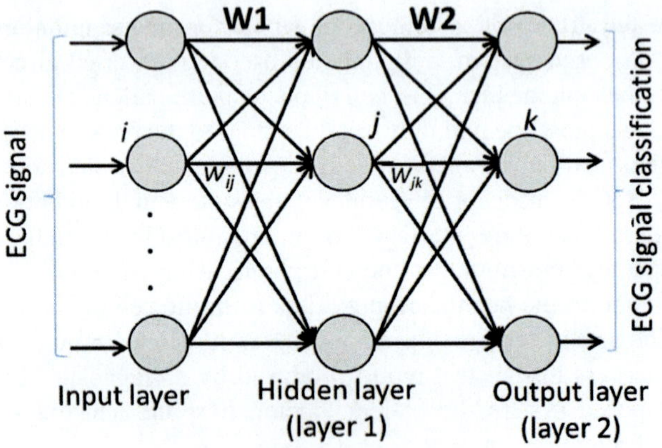

Fig. 2. Block diagram of the FNN.

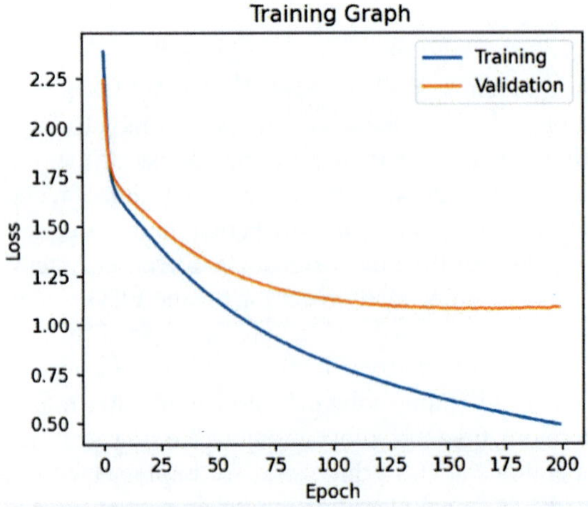

Fig. 3. Training Graph (after 200 epoch the classification error was significantly reduced).

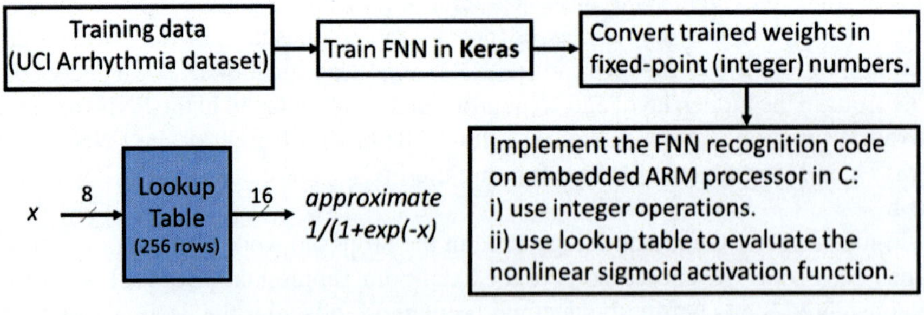

Fig. 4. The methodology used for the fixed-point implementation of the FNN.

4 Hardware Prototype and Result

4.1 Hardware Prototype Design

We have designed a prototype of the proposed telemedicine system which is shown in Fig. 5. Based on the design we have implemented a prototype hardware of the system which is shown in Fig. 6. Table 1 shows the hardware components used in the prototype. The digital stethoscope used in the proposed system internally has a very sophisticated microphone sensor. It converts heart, lung, bowel sound into electrical signal which is interfaced to the cell phone through the audio jack port. The cost of a single patient unit of the proposed system is about $50.

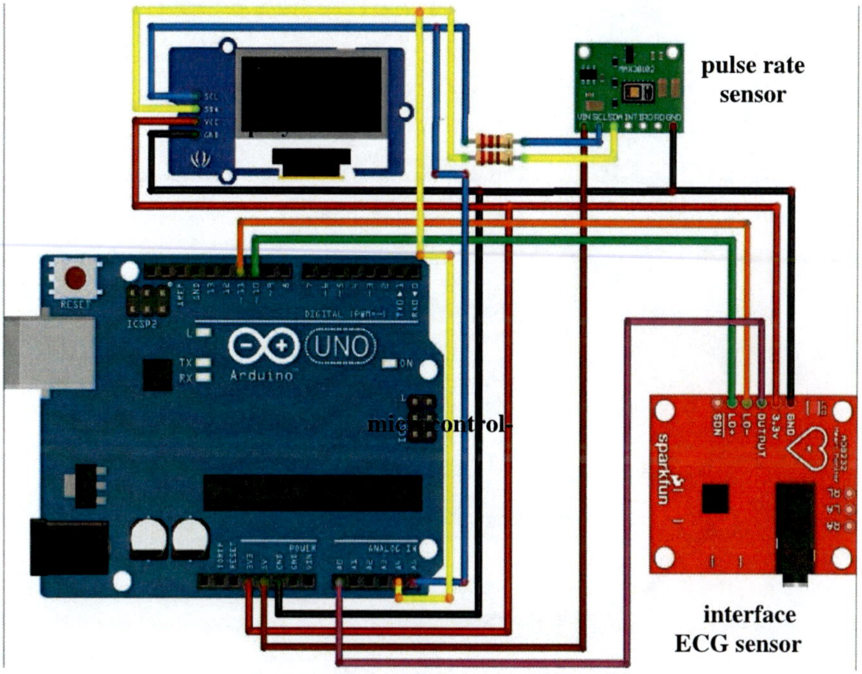

Fig. 5. Prototype hardware diagram.

4.2 ECG Signal Classification Results

In this work, we used an ARM cortex-A57 processor for the fixed-point implementation of the ECG classification FNN. The operating frequency of the processor is 1.43 GHz. Table 2 comparisons the floating-point and fixed-point implementation results. Floating-point model size is 23744 bytes while the integer/fixed-point model size is **11872 bytes** (50% less memory). To classify one ECG signal, the floating-point implementation takes 6.99 us while the fixed-point implementation takes 6.61 us. Hence the proposed fixed-point implementation is 1.06x faster than floating-point implementation. The low energy

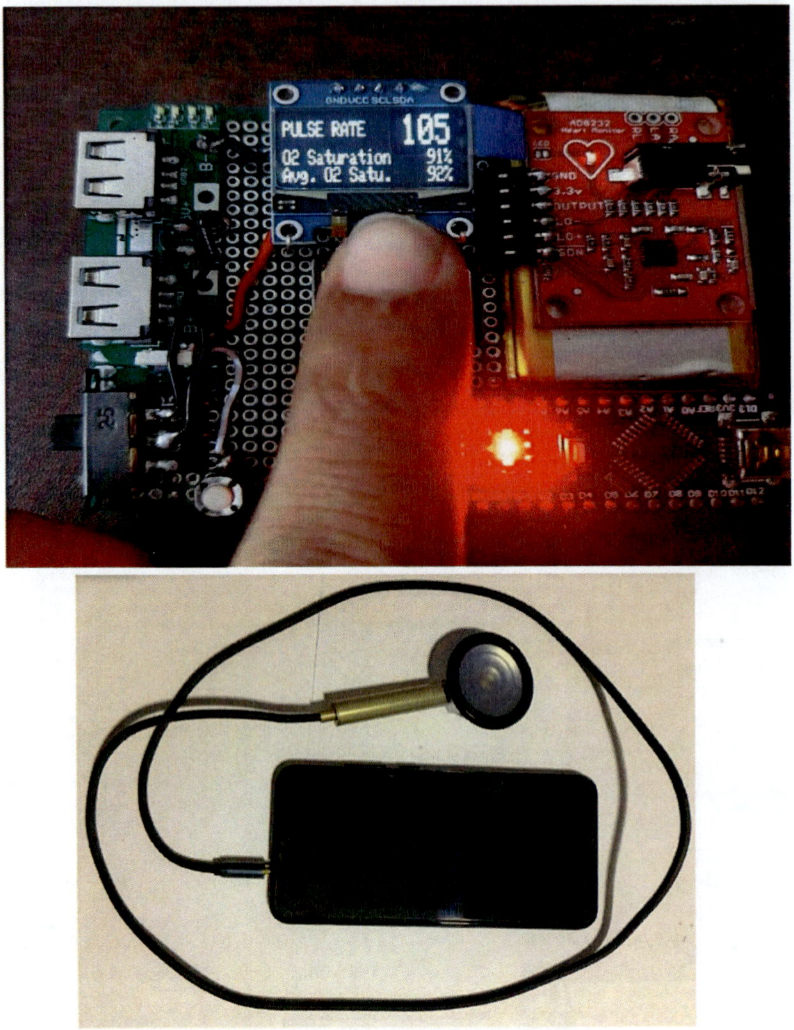

Fig. 6. Prototype hardware implementation.

consumption of the proposed FNN implementation will increase the battery lifetime of the system. Classification accuracy on test dataset is 73% (for both floating-point and the proposed fixed-point implementation).

Table 1. Hardware components used in the prototype.

Component	Use
Arduino-Nano	Read body sensor data
MAX30102	Detect Pulse Rate, SpO_2
AD8232	Detect ECG signal
Bluetooth module	Send sensor data to the cell phone app
Digital stethoscope	Capture heartbeat and lung sound
Cell phone	Receive patient data through Bluetooth and headphone jack

Table 2. Comparison of the floating-point and fixed-point implementations of the FNN for the ECG signal classification task.

	Floating-point implementation	Fixed-point implementation
Accuracy (%)	73	73
FNN model size (byte)	23744	11872
Inference time (μs)	6.99	6.61
Energy consumption for single inference (μJ)	10.485	9.915

5 Conclusion

In the rural areas of Bangladesh people suffer a lot from the lack of proper healthcare and proper medical services. This project will help people from rural areas to get a better healthcare service. Patients will get consultation of specialist doctors remotely. The doctors will be able to examine patients in real-time analyzing multiple body sensor parameters including lung and heart sound. It gives effective and low-cost medical care at home. Single patient side unit of the proposed system costs about $50. The proposed system also has real-time patient monitoring capability based on ECG signal classification. We implemented a FNN for ECG signal classification on an embedded ARM processor using fixed-point operation. To store the FNN model parameters, the proposed implementation requires half of the memory required for a floating-point implementation. In addition to that, the proposed FNN implementation is 1.06x faster than floating-point implementation. Our future work will deploy the system as a pilot project and evaluate the effectiveness of the system based on patient and doctor feedbacks.

References

1. https://bbs.portal.gov.bd/sites/default/files/files/bbs.portal.gov.bd/page/57def76a_aa3c_46e3_9f80_53732eb94a83/2023-04-13-09-35-ee41d2a35dcc47a94a595c88328458f4.pdf
2. Zobair, K.M., Sanzogni, L., Sandhu, K.: Telemedicine healthcare service adoption barriers in rural Bangladesh. Australasian J. Inf. Syst. **24** (2020)

3. Islam, A., Biswas, T.: Health system in Bangladesh: challenges and opportunities. Am. J. Health Res. **2**(6), 366–374 (2014)
4. Albalawi, U., Joshi, S.: Secure and trusted telemedicine in Internet of Things IoT. In: 2018 IEEE 4th World Forum on Internet of Things (WF-IoT), pp. 30–34. IEEE, February 2018
5. Garai, Á., Péntek, I., Adamkó, A.: Revolutionizing healthcare with IoT and cognitive, cloud-based telemedicine. Acta Polytech. Hung **16**(2) (2019)
6. https://www.tytocare.com
7. Alam, M.Z.: MHealth in Bangladesh: current status and future development. Int. Technol. Manage. Rev. **7**(2), 112–124 (2018)
8. Zobair, K.M., Sanzogni, L., Sandhu, K.: Telemedicine healthcare service adoption barriers in rural Bangladesh. Australas. J. Inf. Syst. **24** (2020)
9. Hakim, A.I.: Expected challenges to implement telemedicine service in public hospitals of Bangladesh. J. Soc. Adm. Sci. **3**(3), 231–244 (2016)
10. Chowdhury, S.M., Kabir, M.H., Ashrafuzzaman, K., Kwak, K.S.: A telecommunication network architecture for telemedicine in Bangladesh and its applicability. Int. J. Digit. Content Technol. Appl. **3**(3), 4 (2009)
11. Siddiqua, P., Awal, M.A.: A portable telemedicine system in the context of rural Bangladesh. In: IEEE International Conference on Informatics, Electronics & Vision, pp. 608–611, May 2012
12. Khan, M.M.: IoT based smart healthcare services for rural unprivileged people in Bangladesh: current situation and challenges. In: Presented at 1st International Electronic Conference on Applied Sciences, vol. 10, p. 30, November 2020
13. Zaman, Md.A.U., Sabuj, S.R., Yesmin, R., Hasan, S.S., Ahmed, A.: Toward an IoT-based solution for emergency medical system: an approach to i-medical in Bangladesh. In: Ahad, M.A., Paiva, S., Zafar, S. (eds.) Sustainable and Energy Efficient Computing Paradigms for Society. EICC, pp. 81–105. Springer, Cham (2021). https://doi.org/10.1007/978-3-030-51070-1_5
14. Rahmani, A.M., Babaei, Z., Souri, A.: Event-driven IoT architecture for data analysis of reliable healthcare application using complex event processing. Clust. Comput. **24**, 1347–1360 (2021)
15. Green, M., Ohlsson, M., Forberg, J.L., Björk, J., Edenbrandt, L., Ekelund, U.: Best leads in the standard electrocardiogram for the emergency detection of acute coronary syndrome. J. Electrocardiol. **40**(3), 251–256 (2007)
16. Moons, B., Bankman, D., Verhelst, M.: Embedded deep learning (2019). https://doi.org/10.1007/978-3-319-99223-5
17. Caesarendra, W., et al.: An embedded system using convolutional neural network model for online and real-time ECG signal classification and prediction. Diagnostics **12**(4), 795 (2022)
18. Jeon, T., Kim, B., Jeon, M., Lee, B.G.: Implementation of a portable device for real-time ECG signal analysis. Biomed. Eng. Online **13**(1), 1–13 (2014)
19. Barrois, B., Sentieys, O.: Customizing fixed-point and floating-point arithmetic—a case study in K-means clustering. In: 2017 IEEE International Workshop on Signal Processing Systems (SiPS), pp. 1–6. IEEE (2017)
20. https://archive.ics.uci.edu/ml/datasets/arrhythmia
21. https://keras.io/

Comparison of Predicting Regional Mortalities Using Machine Learning Models

Oğuzhan Çağlar[1] and Figen Özen[2](✉)

[1] Pavotek, Sanayi Mah. Teknopark İstanbul Yerleşkesi, Ar-Ge 4C, Pendik, Istanbul, Turkey
[2] Department of Electrical and Electronics Engineering, Haliç University, Eyüp, Istanbul, Turkey
figenozen@halic.edu.tr

Abstract. Prediction of mortality is an important problem for making plans related to health and insurance systems. In this work, mortality of Africa, America, East Asia and Pacific, Europe and Central Asia, Europe alone, South Asia regions have been studied and predictions are made using fourteen machine learning techniques. These are linear, polynomial, ridge, Bayesian ridge, lasso, elastic net, k-nearest neighbors, support vector (with linear, polynomial and radial basis function kernels), decision tree, random forest, gradient boosting and artificial neural network regressors. The results are compared based on the coefficient of determination and the accuracy values. The best predicting algorithm varies from one region to another. On the other hand, the best accuracy (99.32%) and coefficient of determination (0.9931) are obtained for Africa region and using k-nearest neighbor regressor.

Keywords: Mortality · Machine Learning · Regression · Prediction

1 Introduction

According to [1] there were more than 59.94 million deaths in 2019 all around the World. This number is more than the population of many countries and indeed if all the people who died in 2019 were alive living in a single country in 2023, it would be the 25th most populated country in the World [2]. According to the United Nations' statistics, the population of the World at the beginning of 2019 was 7,724,928,292, and it became 7,804,973,773 at the beginning of 2020 [3]. This means there is an increase in the population. According to the projections made in accordance with the United Nations' medium variant fertility scenario [4] starting from the year 2087, the population of the World will start to decline [5]. Estimating not only births, but also mortality accurately are important for determining sustainable health and economic policies and determining resource allocation to research pertaining to health.

A. Souri and S. Bendak (Eds.): IoTHIC 2023, ECPSCI 8, pp. 59–72, 2024.
https://doi.org/10.1007/978-3-031-52787-6_6

When the literature is surveyed for works on mortality, papers related to different aspects of mortality are found. For example in [6] it is studied how the self perception about one's health at a later age is linked with their mortality. The same question is considered also in the review paper [7]. In [8] to help with the difficult decision to end a life in intensive care unit, a random sample of elderly patients who had to undergo intubation are studied for a 30-day period, and it is concluded that 70% of them die. The same kind of environment is studied in [9] to test the accuracy of forecasting the mortality using Bayesian, naive Bayes networks and extreme gradient boosting. Logistic regression, Gaussian naive Bayes, decision tree, random forest, support vector machine and stack models are created for mortality prediction in the case of heart failure [10]. In [11] the data from 21,732 patients are used to predict mortality using logistic regression. In [12] 39,108 patients are used as subjects to find out 90-day mortality rate after cancer related gastrectomy and it is found that the rate was 8.8%, using machine learning techniques. In [13], lasso, logistic regression methods and extreme gradient boosting are used to predict seven- and thirty-day mortalities after acute heart failure. In [14] random forest, logistic regression, and k-nearest neighbors are used to predict the factors effecting the mortality of children under age five in Ethiopia. The most acceptable results are produced by the random forest model. In [15] regression and tree boosting methods are used to predict the cause of death. In [16] using noninvasive parameters, early mortality prediction is achieved using LightGBM model and with 79.7% accuracy.

Even though some machine learning approaches for predicting mortality can be found in the literature, a study related to predicting regional mortalities is missing. The contributions of this paper are:

- The mortality figures of five different regions of the World, namely Africa, America, East Asia and Pacific, Europe and Central Asia, Europe, and South Asia, are studied and predictions are made based on the available data for the aforementioned regions between 1990–2019.
- Fourteen different machine learning algorithms, namely Linear, Ridge, Bayesian Ridge, Lasso, ElasticNet, Polynomial, Support Vector (with linear, polynomial and radial basis kernel functions), K-Neighbors, Decision Tree, Random Forest, Gradient Boosting and Artificial Neural Network regressors, are employed for prediction of the test values. These methods are selected to sample both classical and contemporary ones.
- The employed methods are compared on the basis of accuracy and coefficient of determination, which are widely accepted metrics for regression problems.

The paper is organized as follows: In Sect. 2 a brief summary of the methods used in the study are provided. In Sect. 3, the metrics for evaluating the performance of the models are introduced. In Sect. 4, experimental works are given. The results are compared for different models and regions on the basis of the performance metrics. In Sect. 5, conclusions are drawn and the future work is mentioned.

2 Methods

In this section, the machine learning methods employed to estimate the time series are described briefly.

2.1 Linear Regression

An elementary technique for estimation is linear regression. It is predicated on the idea that a line can be fitted to the given set of time series. It is incredibly simple to use and only works for straightforward relationships like those in Eq. 1:

$$y_i = b_0 + b_1x_{i1} + b_2x_{i2} + \ldots + b_px_{ip} + e_i \tag{1}$$

where y_i's are the predictions, b_i's are the parameters to be determined, x_{ij}'s are the inputs and e_i's are the errors that are caused by the predictor.

Ridge, Bayesian ridge, lasso, elastic net regressions constitute variants of linear regression where loss functions have slightly different forms.

2.2 Polynomial Regression

Regression using a polynomial rather than a line to fit the data makes it more sophisticated than linear regression. The difficulty of the time series determines the degree of the polynomial and, consequently, the complexity of the fit. Equation 2 provides an explanation for the method:

$$y_i = b_0 + b_1x_i + b_2x_i^2 + \ldots + b_mx_i^m + e_i \; i = 1, 2, \ldots, n \tag{2}$$

where y_i's are the predictions, b_i's are the parameters to be determined, x_i's are the inputs, e_i's are the errors, n is the degree of the polynomial exploited.

2.3 Support Vector Regression

Support vector regression looks for a hyperplane that fits the largest amount of data as in Eq. 3:

$$y = \sum\nolimits_{i=1}^{n} a_i Kernel(x_i, u) + \gamma \tag{3}$$

where x_i's represent the data points, u represents the new data, a_i's and γ represent the parameters, Kernel(x_i,u) represents the kernel function used in the regressor.

Depending on the complexity of the data, different kernel functions can be used to create support vector regressors. For example, the linear kernel is provided by Eq. 4:

$$Kernel(x_i, u) = x_i'u \tag{4}$$

where x_i' represents the transpose of x_i.

Polynomial kernel is defined by Eq. 5:

$$Kernel(x_i, u) = \left(b\left(x_i'u\right) + 1\right)^k \tag{5}$$

where b represents a scaling factor and k represents the degree of the polynomial.

Radial basis kernel is given by Eq. 6:

$$Kernel(x_i, u) = exp\left(-c\|x - u\|^2\right) \tag{6}$$

where c represents a scaling factor [17].

2.4 Decision Tree Regression

Decision nodes and leaves make up a decision tree, and they are built in accordance with the criteria established by the problem. Either a classifier or a regressor can be created using it. It requires careful spatial partitioning and, in this instance, further training to utilize it as a regressor. Figure 1 depicts an illustration of a decision tree structure.

The disadvantage of decision tree model is its susceptibility to overfitting. To overcome this problem, ensemble learning can be used.

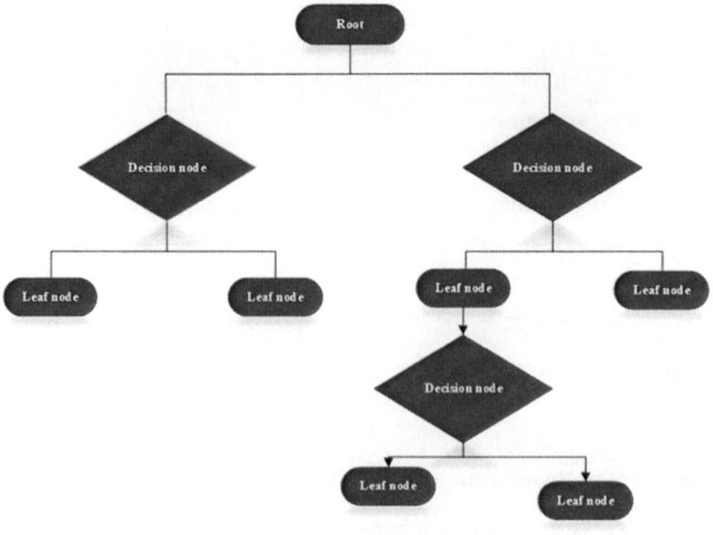

Fig. 1. Structure of a decision tree

2.5 Random Forest Regression

The ensemble learning strategy is used for regression in random forest regression. It integrates predictions from several decision trees in order to produce predictions that are more accurate than those from a single decision tree.

2.6 Gradient Boosting Regression

Gradient boosting is a method for repeatedly combining weak decision tree models so that each new decision tree corrects the inaccuracy of the preceding one, improving the overall performance. Figure 2 illustrates the logic behind gradient boosting mechanism.

2.7 K-Nearest Neighbors Regression

This popular method is nonlinear and relies on the proximity to other samples. No correlation between the features employed and the target variable is needed, which adds flexibility to applications.

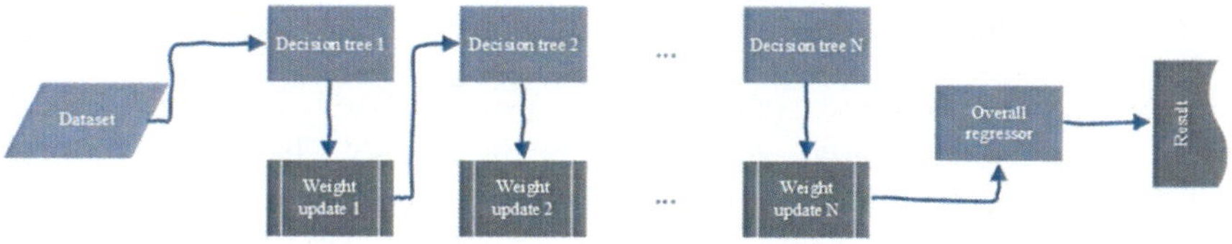

Fig. 2. The operation of gradient boosting regressor

2.8 Artificial Neural Network Regression

Artificial neural networks are created to resemble organic brain networks. They are used to address a variety of issues, including time series estimation, picture recognition, and natural language processing, to mention a few. In Fig. 3, a fundamental artificial neural network is displayed.

When utilizing an artificial neural network to solve a problem, all of the weights must be determined so that the output has the fewest errors possible. Each branch of the neural network is given an unknown weight.

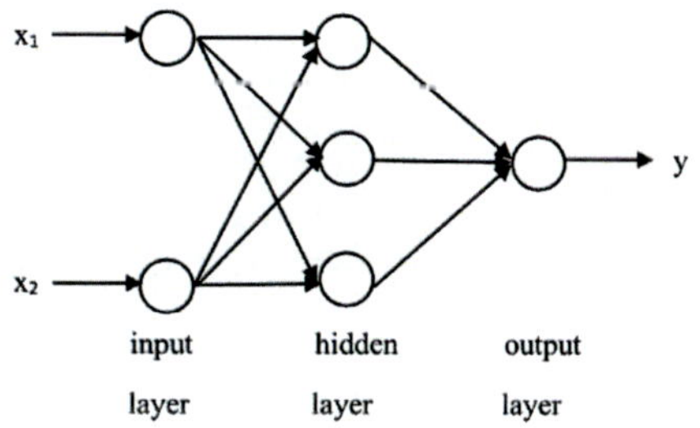

Fig. 3. Simple artificial neural network

3 Performance Metrics

The performance metrics used to evaluate the success of the models developed are the coefficient of determination (r^2 score) and the mean absolute percentage error (mape) values. Accuracy, which is a commonly used metric, can be computed from mape value.

3.1 Coefficient of Determination

It should ideally be between 0 and 1, where 0 indicates no variation around the mean, and 1 indicates complete variation around the mean. Values close to 1 are preferred. Negative r^2 scores are also possible and in that case, the model is not plausible. The formula used to calculate r^2 score is given by Eq. 7:

$$r^2 score = \frac{model\ variance}{true\ variance} \tag{7}$$

3.2 Mean Absolute Percentage Error

Mean absolute percentage error (mape) values range from 0 to 1. The models with mape values closer to 0 are preferred, which means high accuracy. The formula for mape is given by Eq. 8:

$$mape = \frac{1}{N}\sum_{i=1}^{N}\left|\frac{y_i - \hat{y}_i}{y_i}\right| \tag{8}$$

where y_i represents the target value, $\hat{y}_i$ represents the estimated value and N is the number of data points. The accuracy of a model can be calculated by Eq. 9:

$$accuracy = 1 - mape \tag{9}$$

4 Experiments and Discussion

The data is taken from the public source [1] and split into training and test subsets. The data spans the mortality values between 1990–2019. Seventy per cent of data (21 years) is used for training and the remaining 30% (9 years) is used for test. As far as the experiments are concerned, 14 different regressors are used for mortality prediction.

Figure 4 shows the mortality in Africa. In order to decide which model works better, r^2 scores and mape values also have to be taken into account. Figure 5 shows these values. If Figs. 4 and 5 are compared, it is easily seen that not all of the models in Fig. 4 are depicted in Fig. 5. This is due to the fact that even though models may seem to create reasonable results as far as the prediction charts are concerned, the calculated r^2 scores turn out to be unacceptable. For example support vector models with linear kernel (−0,0493) and polynomial kernel (−0.4608), and Bayesian ridge regressor (−0.0245) have negative values, and thus are unacceptable as models although their mape values are reasonable (8.0782, 8.8816 and 8.0645, respectively). In the discussion that follows, the models with negative r^2 scores are not depicted in r^2 score and mape charts.

To create a successful model, a high r^2 score and a low mape value would be preferred. The highest r^2 value is obtained by k-nearest neighbors regressor (0.9931) and the least mape value (0.6759) is created by the same regressor. Therefore, mortality in Africa is best predicted by k-nearest neighbors regressor (k = 3).

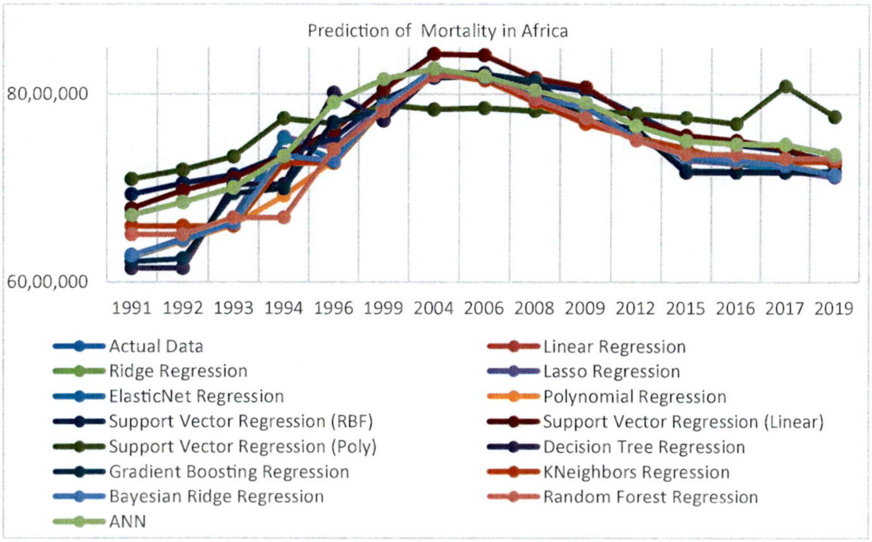

Fig. 4. The mortality in Africa

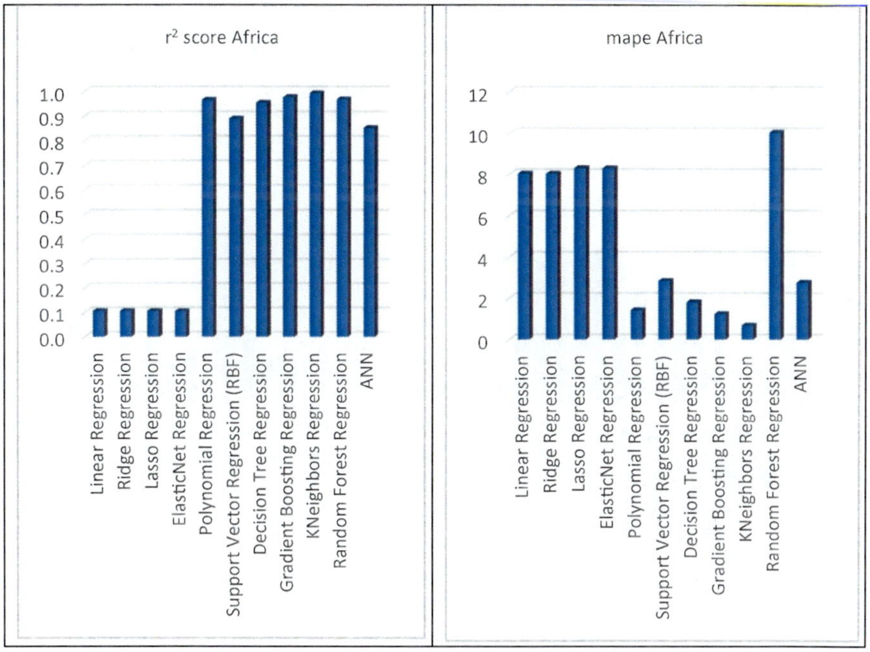

Fig. 5. The performance metrics for Africa

Figure 6 shows the mortality in America. Figure 7 shows r^2 scores and mape values.

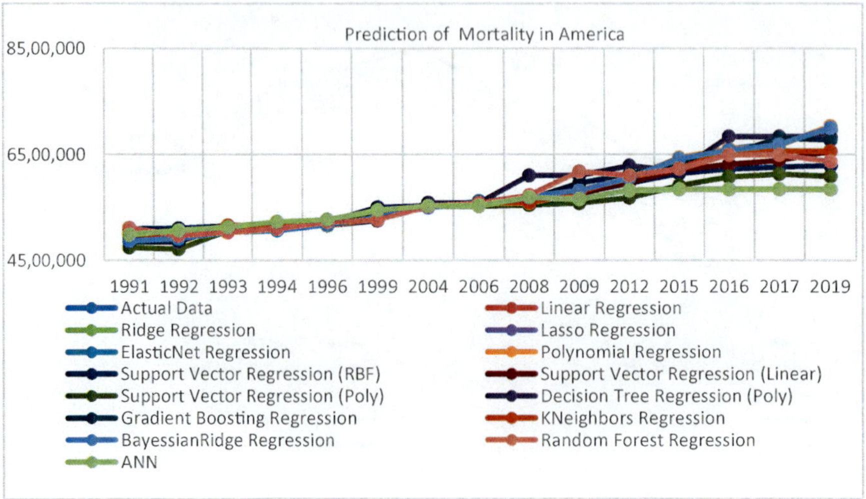

Fig. 6. The mortality in America

The highest r^2 value for America is obtained by polynomial regressor (0.9958) and similarly the least mape value (0.7150) is obtained by the same regressor. Therefore, mortality in America is predicted best by polynomial regressor (degree = 6).

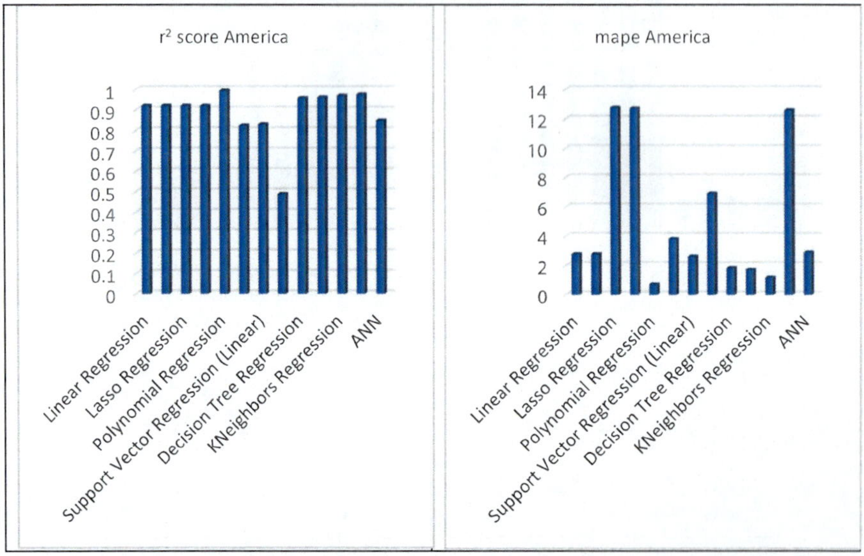

Fig. 7. The performance metrics for America

Figure 8 shows the mortality in East Asia and Pacific. Figure 9 shows r^2 scores and mape values.

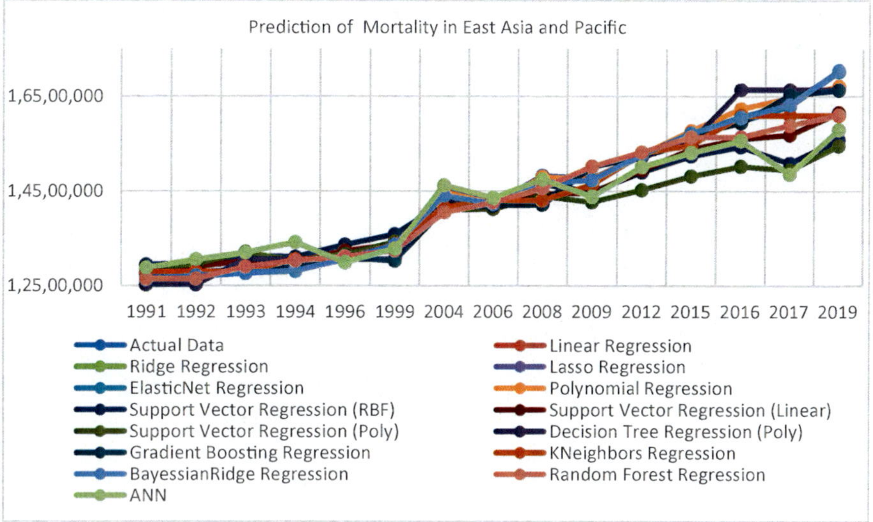

Fig. 8. The mortality in East Asia and Pacific

The highest r^2 value for East Asia and Pacific is obtained by polynomial regressor (0.9848) and similarly the least mape value (0.7832) is obtained by the same regressor. Therefore, mortality in East Asia and Pacific is predicted best by polynomial regressor (degree = 6).

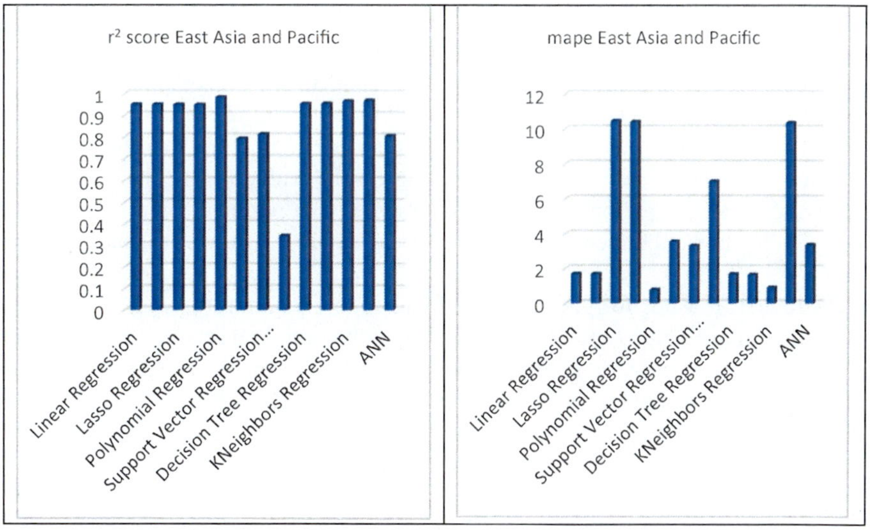

Fig. 9. The performance metrics for East Asia and Pacific

Figure 10 shows the mortality in Europe and Central Asia. Figure 11 shows r^2 scores and mape values.

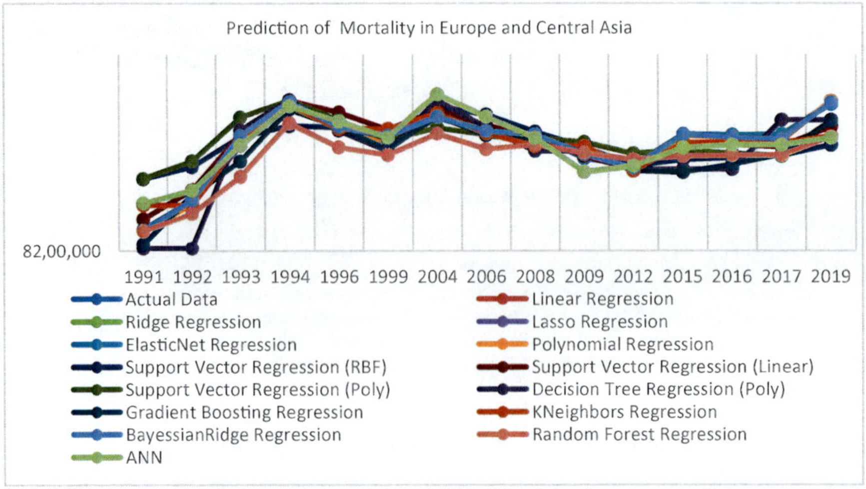

Fig. 10. The mortality in Europe and Central Asia

The highest r^2 value for Europe and Central Asia is obtained by polynomial regressor (0.8392) and the least mape value (0.9109) is obtained by the same regressor. Therefore, mortality in Europe and Central Asia is predicted best by polynomial regressor (degree = 6). The coefficient of determination for this region is not as high as the previous regions considered.

Figure 12 shows the mortality in Europe. Figure 13 shows r^2 scores and mape values.

The highest r^2 value for Europe is obtained by polynomial regressor (0.8470) and the least mape value (0.9053) is created by the same regressor. Therefore, mortality in Europe is predicted best by polynomial regressor (degree = 6). The coefficient of determination for this region is not as high as some other regions.

Figure 14 shows the mortality in South Asia. Figure 15 shows r^2 scores and mape values.

The highest r^2 value for South Asia is obtained by random forest regressor (0.9298) and the least mape value (1.0316) is created by polynomial regressor. To decide which method to choose, another metric, namely root-mean-square error (rmse) value is calculated for both models, where the rmse value is defined by Eq. 10:

$$rmse = \sqrt{\frac{\sum_{i=1}^{N}\left(y_i - \hat{y}_i\right)^2}{N}} \tag{10}$$

where y_i represents the target value, $\hat{y}_i$ represents the estimated value and N is the number of data points The random forest model regressor yields an rmse value of 125436.2574 and the polynomial regressor model yields 140255.0173. Two out of 3 metrics indicate

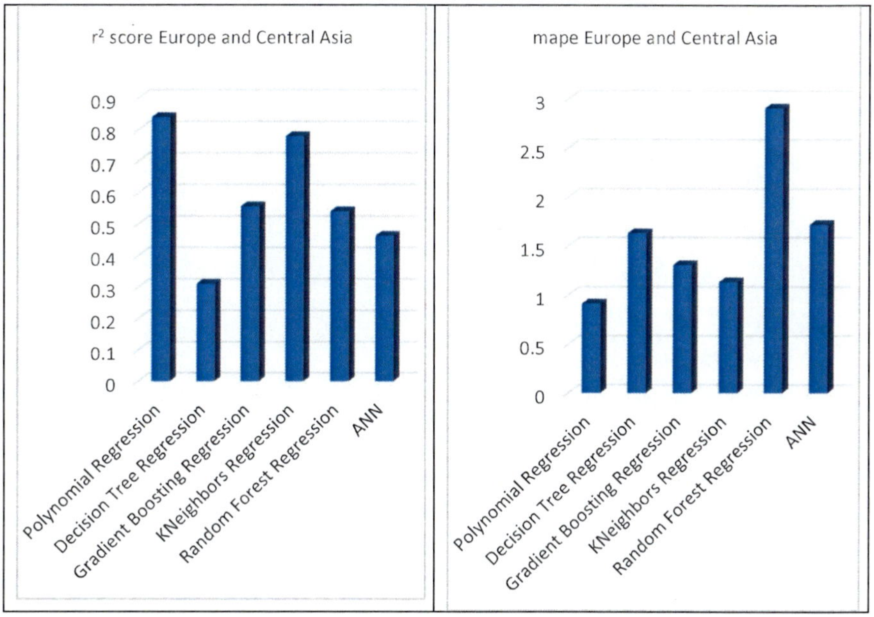

Fig. 11. The performance metrics for Europe and Central Asia

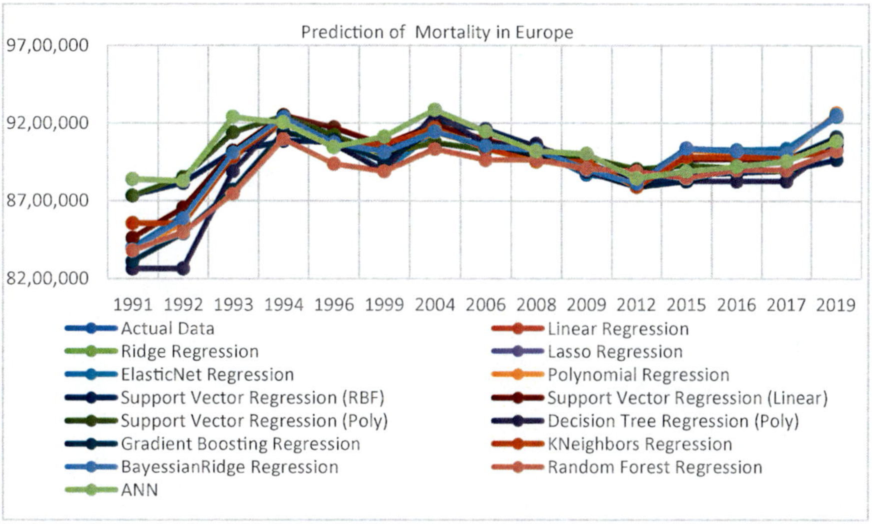

Fig. 12. The mortality in Europe

that random forest (number of estimators = 5) provides a better model for the prediction of mortality in South Asia, and hence it is selected as the best model.

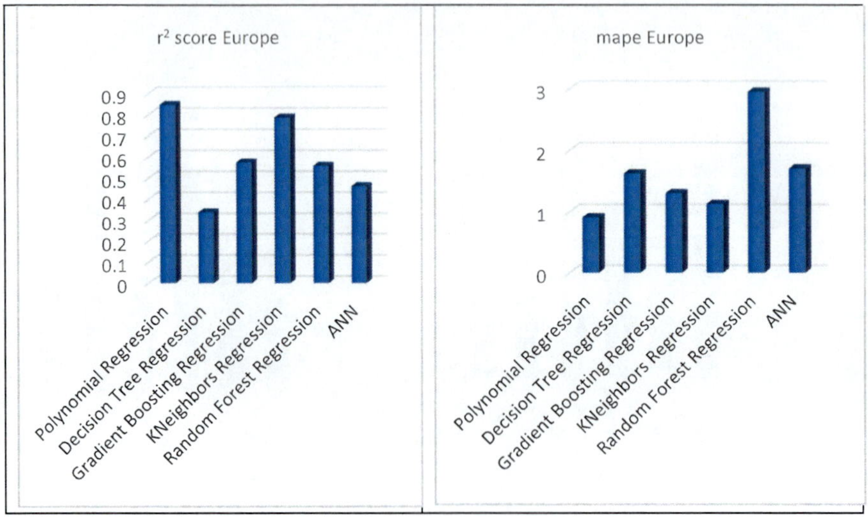

Fig. 13. The performance metrics for Europe

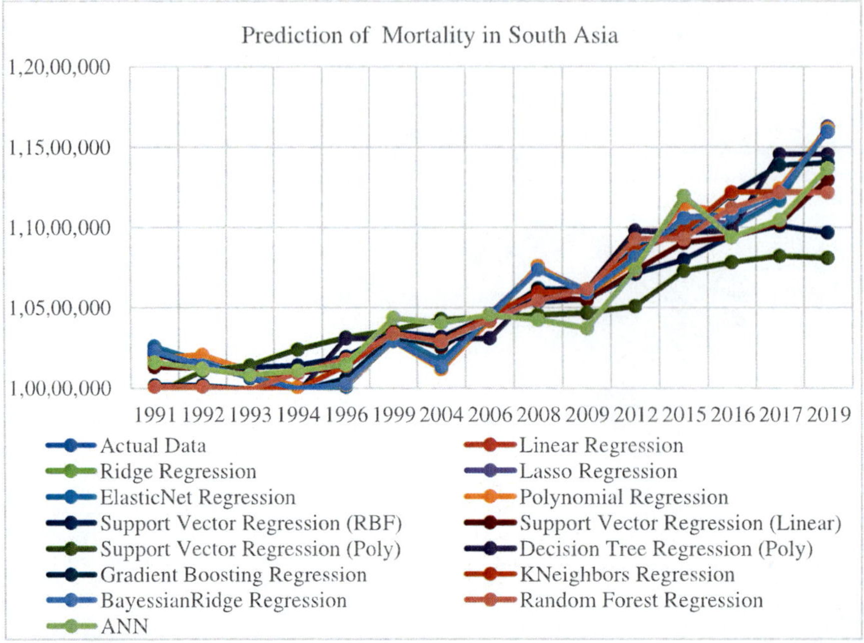

Fig. 14. The mortality in South Asia

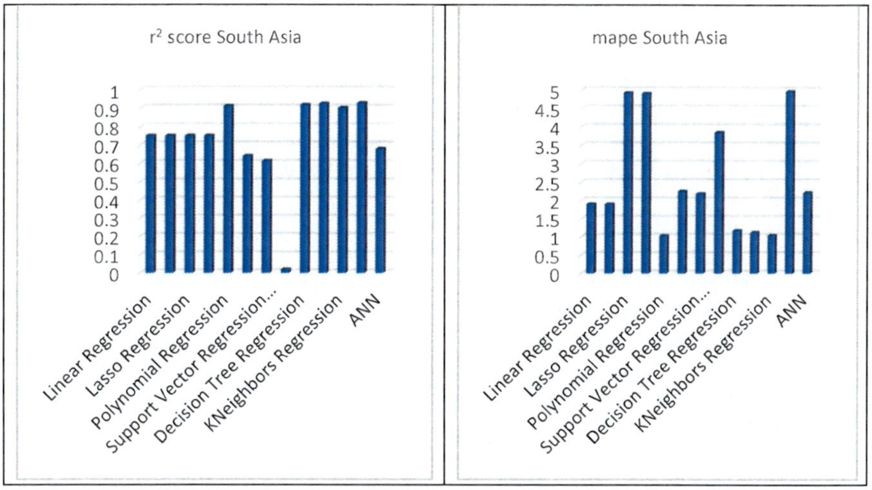

Fig. 15. The performance metrics for South Asia

In the above simulations, Intel Core i7-9750HF processor with 16 GB of RAM and NVIDIA GeForce GTX 1650 graphics card was used. The programs were written using Python programming language in Anaconda environment, exploiting Pandas, Numpy, Matplotlib, Scikit-learn libraries.

5 Conclusion

In this study, the mortality for various regions of the World have been predicted using fourteen machine learning methods. The best results are obtained for Africa region, using a 3-nearest neighbor regressor. The mortality in Africa has been predicted with an accuracy of 99.32%. The mortality in America has been predicted with an accuracy of 99.29%. The accuracy of prediction of East Asia and Pacific is close to this value (99.22%). The accuracy of prediction of Europe and Central Asia and Europe alone are almost the same (99.09%). Finally, the mortality in South Asia has been predicted with an accuracy of 98.97%.

It can be concluded that even though only a 30-year span has been used, the results obtained are satisfactory. Machine learning methods can be used effectively and efficiently to predict variables related to population and health, such as mortality.

In the future, it is planned to estimate the causes of mortality for different parts of the World and make a projection. This intended study could be helpful for future plans of governments and insurance systems.

References

1. our world in data. https://ourworldindata.org/grapher/number-of-deaths-per-year. Accessed 28 July 2023

2. worldometers. https://www.worldometers.info/world-population/population-by-country. Accessed 28 July 2023
3. population UN data. https://population.un.org/wpp/Download/Standard/Mortality. Accessed 28 July 2023
4. U. Nations, D. of Economic, S. Affairs, and P. Division: World Population Prospects 2022: Methodology of the United Nations population estimates and projections (2022). www.unpopulation.org
5. our world in data death-birth. https://ourworldindata.org/grapher/births-and-deaths-projected-to-2100?time=earliest..2100. Accessed 28 July 2023
6. Mossey, J.M., Shapiro, E.: Self-rated health: a predictor of mortality among the elderly. Am. J. Public Health **72**, 800–808 (1982)
7. Idler, E.L., Benyamini, Y.: Self-rated health and mortality: a review of twenty-seven community studies. J. Health Soc. Behav. **38**, 21 (1997)
8. Maley, J.H., Wanis, K.N., Young, J.G., Celi, L.A.: Mortality prediction models, causal effects, and end-of-life decision making in the intensive care unit. BMJ Health Care Inform. **27**(3), e100220 (2020). https://doi.org/10.1136/bmjhci-2020-100220
9. Nistal-Nuño, B.: Developing machine learning models for prediction of mortality in the medical intensive care unit. Comput. Methods Programs Biomed. **216**, 106663 (2022). https://doi.org/10.1016/j.cmpb.2022.106663
10. Kedia, S., Bhushan, M.: Prediction of mortality from heart failure using machine learning. In: 2022 2nd International Conference on Emerging Frontiers in Electrical and Electronic Technologies, ICEFEET 2022, Institute of Electrical and Electronics Engineers Inc. (2022). https://doi.org/10.1109/ICEFEET51821.2022.9848348
11. DeSalvo, K.B., Fan, V.S., McDonell, M.B., Fihn, S.D.: Predicting mortality and healthcare utilization with a single question. Health Serv. Res. **40**(4), 1234–1246 (2005). https://doi.org/10.1111/j.1475-6773.2005.00404.x
12. SenthilKumar, G., et al.: Automated machine learning (AutoML) can predict 90-day mortality after gastrectomy for cancer. Sci. Rep. **13**(1) (2023). https://doi.org/10.1038/s41598-023-37396-3
13. Austin, D.E., et al.: Comparison of machine learning and the regression-based EHMRG model for predicting early mortality in acute heart failure. Int. J. Cardiol. **365**, 78–84 (2022). https://doi.org/10.1016/j.ijcard.2022.07.035
14. Bitew, F.H., Nyarko, S.H., Potter, L., Sparks, C.S.: Machine learning approach for predicting under-five mortality determinants in Ethiopia: evidence from the 2016 Ethiopian Demographic and Health Survey. Genus **76**(1) (2020). https://doi.org/10.1186/s41118-020-00106-2
15. Deprez, P., Shevchenko, P.V., Wüthrich, M.V.: Machine learning techniques for mortality modeling. Eur. Actuar. J. **7**(2), 337–352 (2017). https://doi.org/10.1007/s13385-017-0152-4
16. Zhang, G., Xu, J., Yu, M., Yuan, J., Chen, F.: A machine learning approach for mortality prediction only using non-invasive parameters. Med. Biol. Eng. Comput. **58**, 2195–2238 (2020). https://doi.org/10.1007/s11517-020-02174-0/Published
17. Kuhn, M., Johnson, K.: Applied Predictive Modeling. Springer, New York (2016)

Benign and Malignant Cancer Prediction Using Deep Learning and Generating Pathologist Diagnostic Report

Kaliappan Madasamy[1(✉)], Vimal Shanmuganathan[1(✉)], Nithish[1], Vishakan[1], Vijayabhaskar[2], Muthukumar[3], Balamurali Ramakrishnan[4], and M. Ramnath[1]

[1] Deep Learning Lab, Department of Artificial Intelligence and Data Science, Ramco Institute of Technology, Rajapalayam, Tamilnadu, India
kalsrajan@yahoo.co.in, svimalphd@gmail.com, imyadavcodes@gmail.com

[2] Hera Diagnostics, Rajapalayam, Tamilnadu, India
vijay@hera-tech.in

[3] Department of Pathology, Kalasalingam Medical College and Hospital, Krishnankoil, Tamilnadu, India
mkclassroom1617@gmail.com

[4] Centre for Non Linear Systems, Chennai Institute of Technology, Chennai, Tamilnadu, India
balamurali@citchennai.net

Abstract. The genesis of the proposition to employ deep learning methods for the identification of cancer images stems from the pressing need to augment the diagnosis and treatment of cancer, a significant public health concern worldwide. This inquiry postulates the conception of a mechanism that employs artificial intelligence (AI) to prognosticate the presence of benign and malignant cancer, with a particular emphasis on colon and breast cancer. The proposed mechanism uses the CNN model to attain precise detection of these cancer types from medical images. Furthermore, the study seeks to verify clinical reports concerning the existence of malignant and benign tumors. The research also centers on producing pathologist reports utilizing AI, utilizing the YOLOV5 AI model to diminish diagnostic duration for patients. Additionally, a linear regression AI model is utilized for histopathology image analysis, enabling the classification of benign and malignant cancer. The ultimate objective of this research is to equip pathologists to provide prompt and accurate reports, thereby facilitating informed treatment decisions and reducing cancer morbidity and mortality. The model produced demonstrates specialized expertise in the detection of colon and breast cancer, as it has been trained on a substantial dataset and optimized for accurate classification. The evaluation results underscore the efficacy of the proposed approach, with precision achieving 87%, recall reaching 82%, and a mean average precision at 50% IoU of 88%.These results serve as a testament to the model's robust performance in accurately identifying both benign and malignant cancer cases.

Keywords: YOLOV5 · Residual Neural Network · histopathology image · Colon cancer · Breast cancer

A. Souri and S. Bendak (Eds.): IoTHIC 2023, ECPSCI 8, pp. 73–87, 2024.
https://doi.org/10.1007/978-3-031-52787-6_7

1 Introduction

The origin of the concept to use deep learning techniques for identifying cancer images lies at the intersection of several factors. One of the primary motivations for this research is the need to improve cancer diagnosis and treatment, which is a pressing public health issue globally. Cancer is a complex disease that requires accurate and early diagnosis in order to increase the chances of successful treatment. However, traditional diagnostic methods for cancer, such as histopathology, can be time-consuming and require extensive expertise to interpret accurately. Deep-Learning techniques have emerged as a promising approach for improving the accuracy and efficiency of cancer diagnosis. Deep learning algorithms can learn to recognize patterns in large datasets and can be trained to identify cancerous cells and tissues from histopathology images. This is particularly useful because histopathology images contain a wealth of information that is not always visible to the human eye [1]. The use of deep learning for cancer diagnosis has been a topic of research for several years. The first studies in this area focused on using convolution neural networks (CNNs) to analyze histopathology images [19]. CNNs are a type of deep learning algorithm that are particularly well-suited to image analysis tasks, as they can automatically learn to detect features at different levels of abstraction [15]. By training CNNs on large datasets of histopathology images, researchers have been able to achieve high levels of accuracy in detecting cancerous cells and tissues.

However, while CNNs have been successful in many applications, they are not without limitations. One of the main challenges of using CNNs for cancer diagnosis is the need for large amounts of annotated data [22, 23]. Annotated data is data that has been labeled by human experts to indicate the presence or absence of cancerous cells or tissues. This is a time-consuming and expensive process that requires extensive expertise in histopathology. Additionally, CNNs are susceptible to over fitting, which occurs when the model becomes too specialized to the training data and performs poorly on new data. ResNet is a type of CNN that uses residual connections to allow the network to learn more efficiently from very deep architectures. This has been shown to be particularly effective in applications where large amounts of data are available. In addition to improving the accuracy of cancer diagnosis, deep learning techniques have also been used to develop predictive models for cancer outcomes. By analyzing large datasets of patient data, deep learning algorithms can learn to identify patterns and risk factors that are associated with different outcomes. This can help to improve patient care by identifying patients who are at high risk for poor outcomes and developing personalized treatment plans.

The genesis of the idea to use deep learning techniques for identifying cancer images can also be traced to advances in technology [11]. The availability of large datasets of histopathology images, as well as improvements in computing power and storage, have made it possible to train deep learning algorithms on a scale that was previously not possible. Additionally, the development of open-source deep learning frameworks, such as TensorFlow and PyTorch, has made it easier for researchers to develop and test deep learning models for cancer diagnosis. The inception of the notion to use deep learning techniques for identifying cancer images can be traced to a combination of factors, including the need to improve cancer diagnosis and treatment, advances in technology, and the development of sophisticated deep learning architectures [25]. The use of deep learning for cancer diagnosis has the potential to revolutionize the field by improving the accuracy and efficiency of diagnosis and developing predictive models for patient outcomes. However, there are still challenges that need to be addressed, including the need for large annotated datasets and the risk of overfitting.

2 Literature Survey

Cancer detection using histopathology images is a very active area of research in the field of deep learning and medical image analysis. There have been numerous studies and research papers published in recent years that have explored the use of convolutional neural networks (CNNs) and other deep learning models for this task [9]. One of the most popular and successful deep learning architectures for image classification is ResNet (short for "Residual Network"), which was introduced in 2015 by Microsoft Research. ResNet has been used for a wide range of image classification tasks, including cancer detection in histopathology images. In 2019, a team of researchers from the University of California, Berkeley, and UCSF published a study in the journal Nature that used deep learning to analyze histopathology images for cancer detection. The study used a ResNet model and achieved a classification accuracy of 92.5% for breast cancer metastasis detection.

Another study published in the Journal of Pathology Informatics in 2020 used deep learning models, including ResNet, to classify lung cancer histopathology images. The study achieved a classification accuracy of 91.4% and demonstrated the potential of deep-learning models for accurate and efficient cancer detection.

Overall, deep learning-based cancer detection using histopathology images is a rapidly advancing field with many promising developments [16, 17]. While there are still challenges to overcome, such as the limited availability of high-quality annotated datasets and the need for interpretability in model predictions, the potential benefits of these models for improving cancer diagnosis and treatment make this an important area of research. Cancer is a major public health concern in India, with an estimated 1.39 million new cancer cases and 7.8 lakh cancer-related deaths occurring in the country in 2020, according to the National Cancer Registry Programme. Histopathology plays a crucial role in the diagnosis and treatment of cancer, and the use of artificial intelligence (AI) techniques such as deep learning is increasingly being explored to aid in the detection and classification of cancer cells in histopathology images.

There have been several studies and initiatives in India exploring the use of deep learning and other AI techniques [20] for cancer detection using histopathology images. One study published in the journal Medical Image Analysis in 2020 used a deep learning model to classify breast cancer histopathology images with an accuracy of 91.6%. Another study published in the journal Computer Methods and Programs in Biomedicine in 2021 used a convolutional neural network (CNN) to classify gastric cancer histopathology images with an accuracy of 93.1%.

However, despite these promising developments, there are still challenges to be addressed in the application of deep learning and other AI techniques for cancer detection using histopathology images in India. These include issues related to data quality, data privacy, and the need for standardization and validation of AI-based tools. For example, a study published in the Journal of the American Medical Association found that a deep learning algorithm was able to accurately diagnose skin cancer at a level comparable to dermatologists. Another study published in Nature found that a deep learning algorithm was able to accurately identify breast cancer on mammograms.

Despite these promising results, there is still much work to be done in developing and validating deep learning algorithms for cancer diagnosis [9]. One challenge is the need for large datasets of high-quality histopathology images to train these algorithms. Additionally, there is a need for rigorous evaluation and validation of these algorithms to ensure that they are accurate, reliable, and safe for clinical use. In the context of the current status, the intended paper of using deep learning for cancer detection using histopathology images is of great importance. Early detection of cancer [3] is critical in improving survival rates and reducing the economic burden of cancer treatment. In addition, the use of deep learning algorithms for cancer diagnosis has the potential to improve the accuracy and efficiency of cancer diagnosis, leading to better patient outcomes. The envisioned paper of using deep learning for cancer detection using histopathology images is of great importance in the context of the current status of cancer diagnosis and treatment [4, 8]. With the potential to improve the accuracy and speed of cancer diagnosis, deep learning has the potential to revolutionize cancer care and improve patient outcomes. The World Health Organization estimates that cancer is the second leading cause of death globally, accounting for about 10 million deaths in 2020. The use of deep learning algorithms for cancer diagnosis has the potential to reduce the number of unnecessary biopsies and surgeries, which can lead to significant cost savings for patients and healthcare systems. According to a study published in The Lancet, the global economic burden of cancer was estimated to be $1.16 trillion in 2020. The accuracy of histopathology-based cancer diagnosis can vary widely depending on the type of cancer, with reported diagnostic accuracy ranging from 70% to 95%. In a study published in Nature, a deep learning algorithm was able to accurately identify lung cancer on CT scans, with a sensitivity of 94% and a specificity of 93%. The use of deep learning algorithms for cancer diagnosis has the potential to improve access to care for patients in underserved areas, as it can reduce the need for expert pathologists to physically examine tissue samples.

3 Data Sources and Diagnostic Approaches in Cancer Detection

3.1 Places to Get Reliable Data From

The paper focuses greatly on detecting Cancer from Histopathology images. There are several reliable websites where you can find histopathology image datasets for cancer detection using deep learning. Some of these are:

3.1.1 The Cancer Genome Atlas (TCGA)

TCGA provides a comprehensive collection of publicly available cancer genomic and histopathology data. You can download whole slide images (WSI) from the TCGA website for different types of cancers, including breast, lung, colon, and prostate cancer.

3.1.2 The Cancer Imaging Archive (TCIA)

TCIA is a public repository of cancer imaging data. You can find a large number of histopathology images of different cancer types, including breast, lung, and prostate cancer, in the TCIA dataset.

3.1.3 The PatchCamelyon (PCam) Dataset

The PCam dataset contains 327,680 color images of lymph node sections with metastatic tissue. It is specifically designed for training deep learning models for cancer detection.

The dataset for the model is taken from below.

3.1.4 Cancer and Its Types

Cancer is one of the most dreaded diseases of human beings and is a major cause of death all over the globe [9]. More than a million Indians suffer from cancer and a large number of them die from it annually. The mechanisms that underlie development of cancer or oncogenic transformation of cells, its treatment and control have been some of the most intense areas of research in biology and medicine. In our body, cell growth and differentiation are highly controlled and regulated. In cancer cells, there is breakdown of these regulatory mechanisms. Normal cells show a property called contact inhibition by virtue of which contact with other cells inhibits their uncontrolled growth. Cancer cells appears to have lost this property. As a result of this, cancerous cells just continue to divide giving rise to masses of cells called tumors [5].

Tumors are of two types:

- Benign
- malignant

Benign tumors normally remain confined to their original location and do not spread to other parts of the body and cause little damage.

Characteristics of Benign Tumors are described below:

- Cell Growth and Division: Cells in benign tumors typically exhibit controlled and slow growth. They resemble normal cells and maintain their original function.
- Encapsulation: Benign tumors are usually encapsulated within a fibrous capsule that separates them from surrounding tissues. This encapsulation helps restrict their growth and prevents invasion into adjacent tissues.
- Cell Appearance: The cells within benign tumors often closely resemble normal cells under a microscope, with well-defined cell borders and regular nuclei.
- Mitotic Activity: Mitosis, or cell division, is less frequent and orderly in benign tumors compared to malignant tumors.

The malignant tumors, on the other hand are a mass of proliferating cells called neoplastic or tumor cells. These cells grow very rapidly, invading and damaging the surrounding normal tissues. As these cells actively divide and grow, they also starve the normal cells by competing for vital nutrients.

Characteristics of Malignant Tumors are mentioned below:

- Uncontrolled Cell Growth: Cells within malignant tumors divide rapidly and uncontrollably, often forming irregular masses.
- Invasion: Malignant tumor cells have the ability to invade surrounding tissues and structures. They can infiltrate neighboring tissues, blood vessels, and lymphatic vessels.
- Metastasis: The most distinctive feature of malignant tumors is their potential to metastasize. Cells can break away from the primary tumor and travel via the bloodstream or lymphatic system to distant sites, where they establish secondary tumors.

All the above-mentioned characteristics are clearly visible and identifiable in the considered dataset below.

3.1.5 Diagnostic Methods for Cancer

Methods for diagnosing cancer, and the specific method used will depend on the type of cancer and the individual's symptoms. Some of the most common methods of cancer diagnosis include:

Biopsy: This is the most reliable way to diagnose cancer. A small sample of tissue is removed from the affected area and examined under a microscope for abnormal cells.

Imaging tests: These include X-rays, CT scans, MRI scans, and PET scans. These tests can help identify tumors and determine the size and location of the cancer.

Endoscopy: This involves inserting a thin, flexible tube with a camera into the body to examine the inside of organs or tissues.

Molecular testing: This is a type of testing that looks for changes in the DNA or other molecules that are specific to certain types of cancer.

4 Methodology

4.1 Proposed System

Our model is specifically designed to deal with colon and breast cancer images only. This means that it has been trained on a large dataset of images of these two types of cancer, and it has been optimized to accurately classify new images as either colon or breast cancer. The model has been developed using advanced machine learning techniques, including deep learning algorithms [12], which allow it to analyze complex patterns and features in the images that are characteristic of each type of cancer. By focusing exclusively on these two types of cancer, our model is able to achieve a high degree of accuracy in its predictions and provide valuable insights into the diagnosis and treatment of colon and breast cancer. While our model may not be suitable for detecting other types of cancer, its focused approach allows it to excel in its specific domain, making it a valuable tool for researchers, clinicians, and patients alike.

4.1.1 ResNet Approach

ResNet152V2 is a convolutional neural network (CNN) model [14] that has been pre-trained on a large dataset of images called ImageNet. It is a variant of the original

ResNet model, which was introduced to address the problem of vanishing gradients in very deep neural networks. ResNet152V2 is a very deep neural network that contains 152 layers, and it has shown to be effective in a wide range of image classification tasks. The ResNet152V2 model is known for its ability to extract high-level features from images, which makes it an excellent choice for transfer learning applications. Transfer learning involves using a pre-trained model as a starting point for a new task, rather than training a new model from scratch. By utilizing the pre-trained ResNet152V2 model, it is possible to achieve high accuracy on image classification tasks related to colon and breast cancer with relatively few training examples. In our Model 2 we have used RESNET with a transfer learning approach. In our RESNET model we do not split the data into train and test. Instead, we just use deep transfer learning approach and make the model even easier to work. The code defines and trains a machine learning model called ResNet model that can identify colon and breast cancer in images.

The pre-trained model part of the code imports a pre-trained model called ResNet152V2, which has already learned how to identify many different objects in images. The code then adds a few layers to the ResNet152V2 model to "fine-tune" it for the specific task of identifying colon and breast cancer. The compile function of the model specifies the optimizer, loss function, and evaluation metric to be used during training. The fit function [24] trains the model on the provided training data for a certain number of epochs (here, 10). The model's performance on a separate validation dataset is evaluated during training, and the training history is recorded. The goal of this code is to train a model that can accurately identify colon and breast cancer from images. By doing so, this model could potentially assist in the early detection and treatment of these types of cancers related to colon and breast cancer with relatively few training examples.

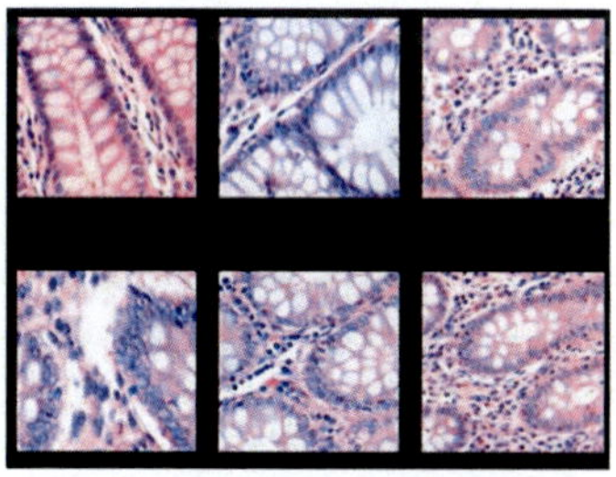

Fig. 1. Benign Samples

After the complete building of a model, we were able to find few insights from the cancer cells which are listed below:

1. Cells are looking tightly packed in slides annotated as 'adenocarcinoma'
2. Cells are loosely packed in slides annotated as 'benign' (Fig. 1).

Before being sampled to increase their scale, histopathological was reduced in size to 224 × 224. Affine image transformations such as rotation, translation, scaling [26] (zoom in/out), and inversion were then coupled to provide new information. Batch normalization [13] was employed both before and after each activation and convolution.

Also, the batches ranged in size from 40 to 80. The model was trained for 15 rounds. The parameters epsilon (at 0.001), momentum (at 0.99), and weight decay (at 0.0001) were adjusted. The error rate plateaued after an initial learning rate of 0.001. There was a 0.5 decrease in the learning rate. Only 10% of the photos in the dataset were utilized for testing and validation, whereas 90% were used for training. In order to get the best outcomes, we applied a number of hyper-parameter techniques, such as regularization and optimization using the AdaMax and SGD optimizers and the categorical cross-entropy loss function. The optimal values for all of the tested model's hyper-parameters [27] are shown in Table 1 (Fig. 2).

Table 1. Resnet Parameter Values

Parameters	Value	Best value
No of Epoches	16	16
Batch size	40/80	80
Activation	ReLU	ReLU
Dropout	0.8	0.7
Loss	10	10

After the training and testing we are comparing the Train and Validation loss with respect to the Epoch taken to run which is shown the following Fig. 3. We are here able to observe that as we increase the number of Epochs the loss is minimized and the Accuracy is increased.

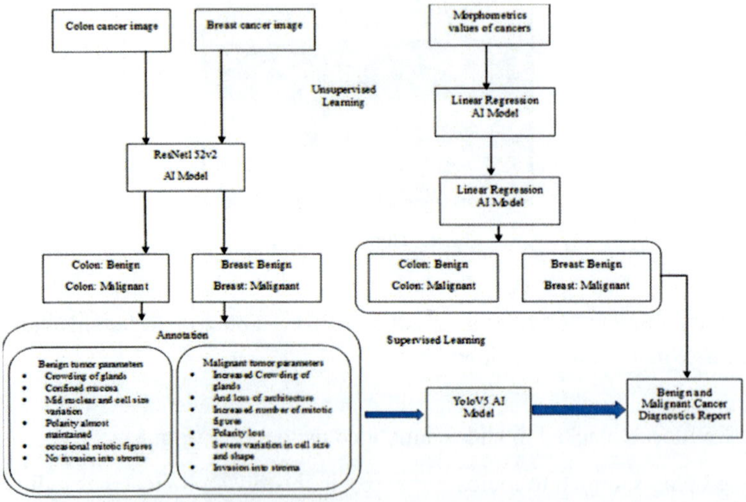

Fig. 2. Conceptual flow diagram of Cancer prediction

4.1.2 The Linear Regression Approach

The next approach that we are going to deal with is the linear regression approach. In this linear regression approach, we take a data set with a few parameters which could determine cancer of any type. Initially in this approach we take only 10 parameters for the analysis. Then after we develop the parameters to account of 30 by including the standard error and the worst value. By doing so, we are capable of increasing the accuracy of the model to higher extent. With this approach we are able to get an accuracy of 92% for training data set and 90% data set.

The parameters that we have taken in here are listed below:

- "Radius mean",
- "Texture mean",
- "Perimeter mean",
- "Area mean",
- "Smoothness mean",
- "Compactness mean",
- "Concavity mean",
- "Concave points mean",
- "Symmetry mean",
- "Fractal dimension mean",
- "Radius se",
- "Texture se",
- "Perimeter se",
- "Area se",
- "Smoothness se",
- "Compactness se",
- "Concavity se",
- "Concave points se",
- "Symmetry se",
- "Fractal dimension se",
- "Radius worst",
- "Texture worst",
- "Perimeter worst",
- "Area worst",
- "Smoothness worst",
- "Compactness worst",
- "Concavity worst",
- "Concave points worst",
- "Symmetry worst",
- "Fractal dimension worst"

The goal of linear regression is to estimate the values the sum of squared errors (SSE) between the predicted values and the actual values of the output variable. This is typically done using a method called least squares, which involves finding the values of the coefficients that minimize the sum of the squared differences between the predicted and actual values of y.

However, they also have limitations, such as their sensitivity to outliers and the assumption of linearity between the input and output variables. As such, it is important to carefully evaluate the assumptions and limitations of linear regression models before using them for predictive modelling [21].

4.1.3 The Labelling Approach Using Annotations on the Histopathology Images

In this approach, we label the images using labelling tools and then use it in their model. We progress on to this approach because the unsupervised method was not able to talk about the reason why the cell is cancerous. But in this approach, we would try to get the reason for the cancer cell being cancerous. The reliable parameters on which they sell is classified as cancerous or benign is listed below:

a. Cell polarity:
   In cancer cells, the nucleus polarity is always lost.
b. Cell size and shape:
   Cancer cells show huge variation in their cell shape and size.
   Invasion into the stroma:
   The extra or the surplus number of cancerous cells are also found to invade into the stroma.
c. Mitotic figures:
   Abnormal mitotic growths are observed in cancer cells.
d. Nucleus size and shape:
   Cancerous cell shows a huge variation in the nucleus size and shape. The nucleus of cancer cells seems to be very charged and distorted.
e. Chromatin content - Normal or Hyperchromatic
   Loss of normal architecture-
f. Increased Nuclear cytoplasmic ratio:
   Now in this approach we trained our model based on the listed parameters and we train it to deliver the possible reason for cancer with the output. By these parameters we were also able to observe few other points.
g. Benign tumors showed all these below listed properties:
   - Crowding of glands
   - Confined to Mucosa
   - Mild Nuclear and cell size and shape variation
   - Polarity almost maintained
   - Occasional Mitotic figures
h. Malignant tumors showed these properties varied to the benign ones:
   - Increased crowding of glands and loss of architecture
   - Increased number of Mitotic figures
   - Polarity lost
   - Severe variation in cell size and shape
   - Invasion into stroma

The YOLOv5 model is a state-of-the-art object detection model that is designed to accurately and efficiently detect objects in real-time images and videos. It is an upgrade to previous YOLO versions, with better performance, speed, and accuracy. The YOLOv5 model is based on a deep neural network architecture, which is trained on a large dataset of labeled images [18]. During training, the model learns to identify and classify objects in images, as well as predict their location and size. This allows the model to accurately detect objects of different shapes, sizes, and orientations, even when they are partially occluded or in cluttered environments. The YOLOv5 model uses a single-stage object detection approach, which means that it directly predicts the bounding boxes and class probabilities for all objects in an image in a single pass. This is in contrast to two-stage approaches, which first generate region proposals and then classify them. The YOLOv5 model is designed to be fast and efficient, with inference times of just a few milliseconds per image on a typical GPU. This makes it well-suited for real-time applications such as video surveillance, robotics, and autonomous vehicles.

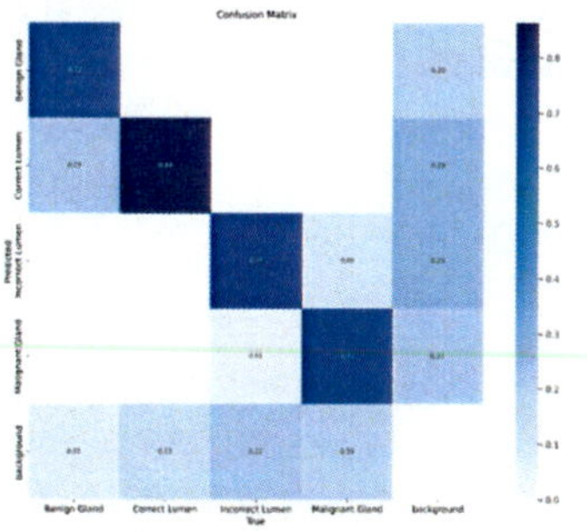

Fig. 3. Confusion matrix

The Cancer Cell detection model which where we used an annotated dataset of types of cells in the Histopathology same, we were able to train a YOLOv5 model with an very good accuracy. When we ran the test inference the model was able to produce the following result.

Precision-confidence curve (PRC) is a graphical plot of the precision and confidence of a binary classifier for different thresholds. The precision is the fraction of positive predictions that are actually positive, while the confidence is the probability that a positive prediction is correct. PRCs are used to evaluate the performance of binary classifiers, especially when the classes are imbalanced.

The final accuracy metrics from the Tensor Board looked like the following had had precision above 86% and the other important accuracy metrics are also displayed. Precision and recall are two important metrics used to evaluate the performance of machine learning models in healthcare. Precision measures the fraction of positive predictions that are actually positive, while recall measures the fraction of actual positives that are predicted as positive. In healthcare, precision is often more important than recall. This is because false positives can have serious consequences, such as unnecessary tests or treatments. Recall is also important in healthcare, especially for diseases that are rare or difficult to diagnose. For example, a model that predicts that a patient has a rare disease with high recall will be more likely to identify patients who actually have the disease, even if it also misses some patients who do have the disease. The choice of which metric is more important depends on the specific application. In general, precision is more important when false positives are more serious than false negatives, and recall is more important when false negatives are more serious than false positives.

Use of Precision in our case: (Predicting cancer) A model that predicts that a patient has cancer with high precision will be less likely to miss a cancer diagnosis, even if it also predicts that some patients who do not have cancer have cancer. This is important because false positives can have serious consequences, such as unnecessary tests or treatment.

Precision is the fraction of predicted bounding boxes that are correctly classified. Recall is the fraction of ground-truth bounding boxes that are correctly classified. Mean Average Precision (mAP) is a measure of the overall performance of an object detection model. The evaluation results underscore the efficacy of the proposed approach, with precision achieving 87%, recall reaching 82%, and a mean average precision at 50% IoU of 88%.These results serve as a testament to the model's robust performance in accurately identifying both benign and malignant cancer cases.

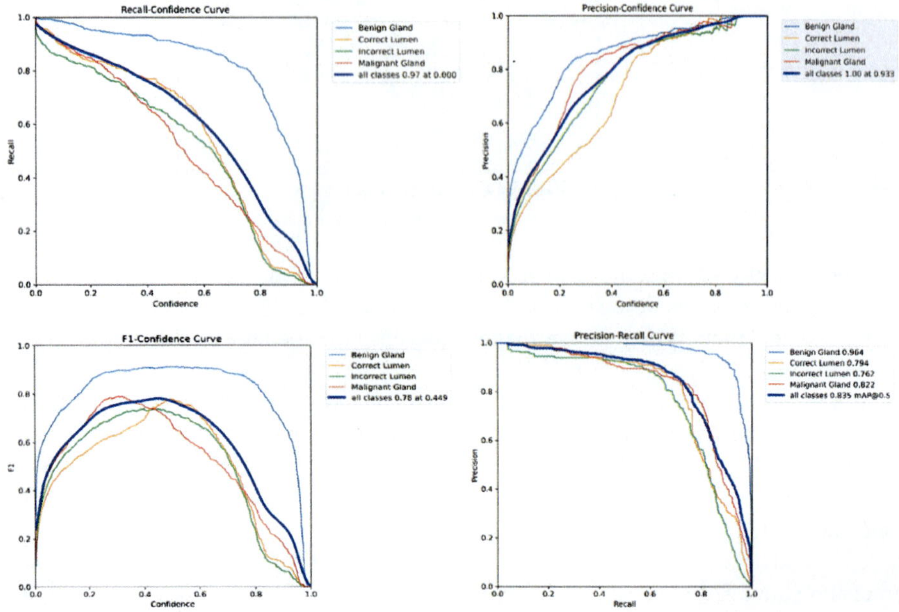

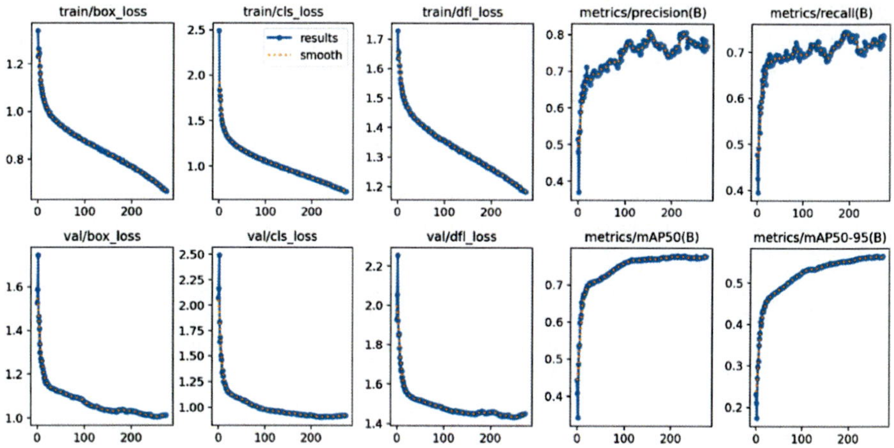

5 Conclusion

The proposition to employ deep learning methods for the identification of cancer images, with a particular focus on colon and breast cancer, emerges from the urgent need to enhance cancer diagnosis and treatment. By utilizing advanced artificial intelligence techniques, such as the CNN model, the proposed mechanism aims to accurately detect and predict the presence of benign and malignant cancer. The research also addresses the authentication of clinical reports, expedites the generation of pathologist reports using AI, and enables histopathology image analysis for precise classification of cancer types. Comparing the proposed CNN model with other state-of-the-art models would involve; Architectural Choices: Different CNN architectures might be chosen based on the complexity of the problem and the available data. State-of-the-art architectures like ResNet, Inception, and DenseNet have demonstrated improved performance by addressing issues like vanishing gradients and information bottleneck.; Transfer Learning: Many state-of-the-art models leverage pre-trained networks on large image datasets (ImageNet) and then fine-tune them for specific tasks like cancer detection. This transfer learning approach can significantly improve performance, especially when the dataset for the specific task is limited.; Ensemble Methods: Combining predictions from multiple models or different versions of the same model can lead to improved accuracy and robustness.; Computational Resources: Some state-of-the-art models may require more computational resources for training and inference, which can impact their practicality in real-world applications. The ultimate goal is to empower pathologists to provide timely and accurate reports, leading to informed treatment decisions and a reduction in cancer morbidity and mortality. Future directions might be briefed as; Multi-Cancer Integration: Extend research to diverse cancer types, creating a multi-cancer model. Fuse data from various sources, like radiology and genomics, for comprehensive diagnostics; Explainable AI (XAI): Improve model transparency by developing methods that clarify its decision rationale. Boost trust among pathologists and clinicians, refining accuracy while enhancing understanding of AI-generated conclusions.

Acknowledgement. Here, I need convey my sincere thanks to Deep Learning Laboratory, Department of Artificial Intelligence and Data Science, Ramco Institute of Technology Tamilnadu, India & Hera Diagnostic Centre, Rajapalayam, Tamilnadu, India.

References

1. Roy, P.S., Saikia, B.J.: Cancer and cure: a critical analysis. Indian J. Cancer **53**(3), 441–442 (2016)
2. Torre, L.A., Siegel, R.L., Ward, E.M., Jemal, A.: Global cancer incidence and mortality rates and trends–an update. Cancer Epidemiol. Biomark. Prev. **25**(1), 16–27 (2016)
3. Chollet, F.: Xception: deep learning with depthwise separable convolutions. In: Proceedings of the 30th IEEE Conference on Computer Vision and Pattern Recognition, CVPR 2017, Honolulu, HI, USA, pp. 1251–1258, July 2017
4. Sadiq, M.T., Akbari, H., Rehman, A.U., et al.: Exploiting feature selection and neural network techniques for identification of focal and nonfocal EEG signals in TQWT domain. J. Healthc. Eng. **2021**, 24 pages (2021). Article ID 6283900
5. Ren, S., He, K., Girshick, R., Sun, J.: Faster R-CNN: towards real-time object detection with region proposal networks. IEEE Trans. Pattern Anal. Mach. Intell. **39**(6), 1137–1149 (2017)
6. Zhong, Z., Sun, L., Huo, Q.: An anchor-free region proposal network for Faster R-CNN-based text detection approaches. Int. J. Doc. Anal. Recogn. **22**(3), 315–327 (2019)
7. Vrinten, L.M., McGregor, M., Heinrich, M., et al.: What do people fear about cancer? A systematic review and meta-synthesis of cancer fears in the general population. Psychooncology **26**(8), 1070–1079 (2017)
8. Zoph, B., Vasudevan, V., Shlens, J., Le, Q.V.: Learning transferable architectures for scalable image recognition (2018). https://arxiv.org/abs/1707.07012v4
9. Abbas-Aghababazadeh, F., Mo, Q., Fridley, B.L.: Statistical genomics in rare cancer. Semin. Cancer Biol. **61**, 1–10 (2020)
10. Asif, M., Khan, W.U., Afzal, H.M.R., et al.: Reduced-complexity LDPC decoding for next-generation IoT networks. Wirel. Commun. Mobile Comput. **2021**, 10 pages (2021). Article ID 2029560
11. Junejo, R., Kaabar, M.K.A., Mohamed, S.: Future robust networks: current scenario and beyond for 6G. IMCC J. Sci. **11**(1), 67–81 (2021)
12. He, K., Zhang, X., Ren, S., Sun, J.: Deep residual learning for image recognition. In: Proceedings of the IEEE Computer Society Conference on Computer Vision and Pattern Recognition, Las Vegas, NV, USA, pp. 770–778, June 2016
13. Balajee, S., Hande, M.P.: History and evolution of cytogenetic techniques: current and future applications in basic and clinical research. Mutat. Res./Genet. Toxicol. Environ. Mutagen. **836**(Part A), 3–12 (2018)
14. Parida, S., Sharma, D.: The microbiome and cancer: creating friendly neighborhoods and removing the foes within. Can. Res. **81**(4), 790–800 (2021)
15. Marx, V.: How to follow metabolic clues to find cancer's Achilles heel. Nat. Methods **16**(3), 221–224 (2019)
16. Baust, J.M., Rabin, Y., Polascik, T.J., et al.: Defeating cancers' adaptive defensive strategies using thermal therapies: examining cancer's therapeutic resistance. Technol. Cancer Res. Treatment **17** (2018)
17. Seelige, R., Searles, S., Bui, J.D.: Innate sensing of cancer's non-immunologic hallmarks. Curr. Opin. Immunol. **50**, 1–8 (2018)
18. Dasgupta, M., Nomura, R., Shuck, R., Yustein, J.: Cancer's Achilles' heel: apoptosis and necroptosis to the rescue. Int. J. Mol. Sci. **18**(1), 23 (2017)

19. Sepp, T., Ujvari, B., Ewald, P.W., Thomas, F., Giraudeau, M.: Urban environment and cancer in wildlife: available evidence and future research avenues. Proc. Royal Soc. B Biol. Sci. **286**(1894) (2019). Article 20182434
20. Lichtenstein, V.: Genetic mosaicism and cancer: cause and effect. Can. Res. **78**(6), 1375–1378 (2018)
21. Lecun, Y., Bengio, Y., Hinton, G.: Deep learning. Nature **521**(7553), 436–444 (2015)
22. Huang, G., Liu, G., Van Der Maaten, Z., Weinberger, K.Q.: Densely connected convolutional networks. In: Proceedings of the 30th IEEE Conference on Computer Vision and Pattern Recognition, CVPR 2017, Honolulu, HI, USA, pp. 4700–4708, July 2017
23. Donahue, J., Jia, Y., Vinyals, O., et al.: DeCAF: a deep convolutional activation feature for generic visual recognition. In: Proceedings of the 31st International Conference on Machine Learning, ICML 2014, Beijing, China, pp. 647–655, June 2014
24. Tan, M., Le, Q.V.: EfficientNet: rethinking model scaling for convolutional neural networks (2020). https://arxiv.org/abs/1905.11946
25. Ioffe, S., Szegedy, C.: Batch normalization: accelerating deep network training by reducing internal covariate shift. In: Proceedings of the 32nd International Conference on Machine Learning, ICML 2015, Lille, France, pp. 448–456 (2015)
26. Royston, P., Altman, D.G.: External validation of a Cox prognostic model: principles and methods. BMC Med. Res. Methodol. **13**(1), 33 (2013)
27. Karamanou, M., Tzavellas, E., Laios, K., Koutsilieris, M., Androutsos, G.: Melancholy as a risk factor for cancer: a historical overview. JBUON **21**(3), 756–759 (2016)
28. Dataset link. https://www.cancerimagingarchive.net/histopathology-imaging-on-tcia/

An Integrated Deep Learning Approach for Computer-Aided Diagnosis of Diverse Diabetic Retinopathy Grading

Şükran Yaman Atcı(✉)

Haliç University, 34060 Istanbul, Turkey
sukranatci@halic.edu.tr

Abstract. Diagnosing and screening diabetic retinopathy pose significant challenges in biomedical research. Utilizing the advancements in deep learning, computer-assisted diagnosis has emerged as a potent technique to examine medical images of patients' eyes and detect damage to blood vessels. Nevertheless, the effectiveness of deep learning models has been impeded by factors such as imbalanced datasets, annotation inaccuracies, limited available images, and inadequate evaluation criteria. In this study, addressed these formidable challenges by employing three established benchmark datasets related to diabetic retinopathy. This approach has facilitated a comprehensive assessment of cutting-edge methodologies. As a result of our study, achieved remarkable precision scores: 93% for standard cases, 89% for mild instances, 81% for moderate conditions, 76% for severe stages, and 96% for diabetic retinopathy phases. Notably, conducted a thorough analysis of a hybrid model that integrates Convolutional Neural Network (CNN) analysis with SHapley Additive exPlanations (SHAP) model derivation. Our findings underscore the suitability of hybrid modeling strategies for detecting anomalies in blood vessels through the utilization of classification models.

Keywords: Diabetic Retinopathy · Image Classification · Object detection · Computer-aided diagnosis · Convolutional Neural Network (CNN)

1 Introduction

A well-known chronic condition linked to a startling growth in fatalities globally, diabetes has adverse consequences typically observed in different parts of the human body, especially the retina of the eyes, which can lead to significant vision loss at later stages of diabetic disease. Diabetic Retinopathy (DR) is a disorder in which the eyes are affected due to diabetes [1, 2]. High blood sugar is present in the retina's blood vessels, causing this problematic disorder. According to recent research, between 2012 and 2021, diabetes will impact 642 million adults worldwide by 2040 [3, 4]; to that purpose, one in three people with diabetes will experience DR [5]. Several DR levels have been classified, including stage zero, which denotes no retinopathy.

A. Souri and S. Bendak (Eds.): IoTHIC 2023, ECPSCI 8, pp. 88–103, 2024.
https://doi.org/10.1007/978-3-031-52787-6_8

In contrast, stages one, two and three indicate mild, moderate and severe non-proliferative diabetic retinopathy conditions. However, the proliferative diabetic retinopathy issue is brought on by stage four, a severe and significant stage, respectively [6]. As it may result in various vision-related problems, such as blurriness or blindness, stage four significantly affects the patient's health conditions and daily routines. Thus, early disease detection of DR is essential to preventing the patient's death in this potentially fatal circumstance [7]. In contrast to labor-intensive and time-consuming manual screening, computer-aided diagnosis (CAD) airing for DR offers a streamlined and efficient approach to accelerate the diagnostic process [8]. Early and accurate illness identification would be possible through automated techniques, which may also be conveniently used for population screening. Recent advancements in computing hardware have made it incredibly simple to use machine learning techniques widely, which has been highly advantageous for the biomedical field [4]. As a result, compared to traditional methods, the application of deep learning has significantly improved the diagnosis of DR [9].

This paper aims to comprehensively compare and analyze multiple computer vision techniques to identify the most effective tasks, such as classification, object identification, and segmentation, within the context of multi-class imbalanced datasets for Diabetic Retinopathy (DR). An imbalanced dataset refers to a situation where the occurrence of majority classes significantly outweighs that of minority classes, resulting in skewed classification outcomes that favor the majority [10–12]. Notably, datasets related to diabetic retinopathy are characterized by a highly uneven distribution of classes, which sets them apart from many other real-world biomedical datasets. The focus is on addressing challenges inherent in building learning models for multi-class imbalanced datasets based on samples, given the difficulty in predicting the prevalence of each class within the distribution [13–15]. Additionally, the study delves into selecting appropriate assessment measures to evaluate the performance of various learning models across diverse computer vision tasks. Unlike binary classification, dealing with sample distributions across multiple classes is more intricate. Robust models are crucial for accurately diagnosing diabetes and determining diabetes types through automated classification tasks. Furthermore, identifying anomalies in retinal images through object detection and segmentation techniques is essential for early and precise therapeutic interventions, reducing the risk of severe vision loss [16].

In classification, the aim is to assign a single class label to an image, making it a global labeling task. Object detection, however, involves sparse labeling, where only specific image pixels are labeled. Convolutional Neural Networks (CNNs), extensively utilized across various domains, have significantly expanded the resolution capabilities of most computer vision problems today. The prowess of CNNs stems from their ability to perform automatic feature extraction and classification in a single step, outperforming conventional methods [17]. Giles et al. [18] categorized CNN training into two methods: training from scratch or utilizing pre-trained networks to fine-tune the model on a target dataset. Models trained on a larger dataset comprising millions of images are pre-trained models.

In this study, described a straightforward approach for rating the severity of DR lesions utilizing SHAP by image processing. Numerous earlier studies recommending extremely accurate solutions demand extensive machine learning expertise. It is challenging to create the same or better algorithms to duplicate past methods in various situations accurately. Our methods of evaluating DR and removing residuals from lesions were based on a relatively straightforward idea; therefore, if they are put to practical use, the suggested approaches might be replicated in other surroundings. Furthermore, introduced a novel ensemble system based on CNNs for the automated diagnosis of different stages of DR. Leveraging transfer learning, extracted distinctive features from the numerous retinal lesions visible in fundus images by amalgamating weights from distinct models into a single model. Specifically, a cloned model computes the average of model weights derived during training. These estimated weights are employed to generate features for input to a custom classifier, which then determines the severity of DR. To investigate the attributes contributing to the outcomes of our prediction models, adopted the SHapley Additive exPlanations (SHAP) analysis approach [19, 20]. SHAP analysis assigns positive and negative contributions of each feature (image region) to the ultimate prediction, offering insights into local feature importance for each image in the dataset. Unlike existing feature analysis approaches that assess the extent of features, the SHAP approach assigns a significance value to each component for a particular prediction [21]. For these purposes, demonstrated a hybrid modeling technique to define the DR locations combination between SHAP outputs of the CNN's iterative solutions on human-eye precise accurately. Utilizing the SHAP analysis technique, highlighted regions within fundus images that frequently exhibit signs of DR or represent varying disease stages, depending on the severity of the condition.

2 Background of Literature Resources

The elevation of blood glucose levels resulting from diabetes gives rise to one of the most critical consequences, Diabetic Retinopathy (DR), which can lead to sudden blindness due to retinal damage. In the realm of DR diagnosis, conventional machine-learning (ML) techniques often integrate manually engineered features [23–27]. Numerous surveys have scrutinized these traditional approaches, as highlighted by Zhu et al. [28]. These methodologies encompass mathematical morphology, retinal lesion tracking, deformable models with thresholding, clustering-based and matched filtering models, as well as hybrid approaches [23, 24, 29]. However, the emergence of deep learning algorithms, fueled by extensive datasets and powerful computing resources, has overwhelmingly outperformed traditional hand-engineered methods in various computer vision tasks over recent years. This transformation is particularly evident in the development of automatic computer-aided diagnosis systems for DR, with various deep learning-based algorithms targeting diverse tasks involving the assessment of retinal fundus images.

In DR detection, the fusion of manually designed features with established machine learning (ML) techniques has been a prevailing approach. A multitude of studies have delved into these conventional techniques [30–35]. Notable examples include mathematical morphology, retinal lesion tracking, thresholding combined with deformable models, clustering-based models, matched filtering models, and hybrid methodologies.

Zhu et al. [28] have also categorized DR diagnosis based on the adopted strategies. Arcadu et al. [36] have explored algorithms designed to extract lesion characteristics from fundus scans, encompassing features such as blood vessel area, exudates, hemorrhages, microaneurysms, and texture. Fleming et al. [37] have evaluated the early advancements in exudate detection, while Ting et al. [32, 33] have provided an overview of algorithms for retinal vascular segmentation. Abràmoff et al. [30] and Dashtbozorg et al. [22] have delved into numerous techniques for segmenting the optic disc (OD) and diagnosing glaucoma.

Utilizing manually crafted features demands specialized expertise, and selecting suitable features necessitates exhaustive exploration of all possible alternatives along with time-consuming parameter tuning. Furthermore, methods reliant on hand-engineered features often lack generalizability. Arcadu et al. [36] employed several morphology and segmentation techniques for detecting blood vessels, hard exudates, and microaneurysms, recognizing the significance of blood vessel segmentation ineffective DR detection. They harnessed the Haar wavelet transform for feature extraction and PCA-based feature selection. In their approach, a neural network based on back-propagation was proposed for two-class classifications. Similarly, Shanthi and Sabeenian [38] employed a multilayer perceptron neural network for DR identification. In an automatic exudate detection methodology, the OD segmentation was accomplished using a graph cuts technique.

Many artificial neural network-based techniques often fail to adequately address the challenges of overfitting when dealing with large-scale fundus images. For instance, Raman et al. [39] introduced a five-class classification system encompassing mild, moderate, severe, NPDR, and PDR categories. They combined OD identification for exudate and microaneurysm extraction in DR diagnosis, employing a genetic approach to pinpoint exudates. Junior and Welger [40] utilized the intersection of abnormal blood vessel thickness to identify exudates and other lesions within fundus images. Similarly, Arcadu et al. [36] employed analogous techniques for DR diagnosis, including k-means clustering and a fuzzy inference system.

The necessity for an autonomous Computer-Aided Diagnosis (CAD) system for DR anomaly detection and severity assessment was emphasized by Shanthi and Sabeenian [38]. Subsequent enhancements led to the development of a comprehensive CAD model capable of detecting retinal microaneurysms and exudates, as well as classifying DR data using classifiers such as Support Vector Machines (SVM) or k-Nearest Neighbors [41, 42]. Zhang et al. [43] utilized feature extraction based on discrete wavelet transform to identify DR abnormalities in fundus images. Morphology and texture analysis methods were employed in various studies to identify DR characteristics in colored fundus images, including blood vessels and hard exudates. Gardner et al. [44] achieved accurate DR classification using a neural network based on pixel intensity values, yielding a robust model with an estimation accuracy of over 80% for five-class DR-level classification.

The primary aim of this study is to develop a robust and efficient Computer-Aided Design (CAD) system for Diabetic Retinopathy (DR). Previous studies [45, 46] have explored multiple retinal image processing techniques and their applicability to CAD-based DR screening. Image preprocessing, segmentation of normal and pathological retinal features, as well as DR detection methods, have been highlighted in studies

[31–33, 41]. Notably, Patton et al. [45] conducted a comprehensive review covering image registration, preprocessing, pathological feature segmentation, and various imaging modalities for DR diagnosis. However, none of these studies provided a comparative assessment of recent state-of-the-art machine learning algorithms.

The versatility of deep learning models has catalyzed significant progress in a wide range of biomedical disciplines. This transformative impact extends to fields including musculoskeletal rehabilitation on rectal, breast, cervical, retinal, and lung cancer treatment, where deep learning-based architectures have ushered in notable advancements in biological applications. In the context of our research, our focus centers on harnessing the capabilities of deep learning-based architectures to tackle tasks such as classification, segmentation, and object recognition within datasets pertinent to diabetic retinopathy.

3 Material and Methodology

In the realm of bio-engineering studies focused on image processing technologies, dealing with unbalanced datasets has been a common challenge. In such datasets, the majority classes significantly outnumber the minority classes, resulting in biased classification outcomes that tend to favor the majority classes [10–12]. Moreover, selecting appropriate evaluation measures plays a pivotal role in accurately assessing the performance of various learning models across their respective computer tasks. Effective models are indispensable for precise diabetes diagnosis and classification and detecting of anomalies in retinal images through object detection and segmentation techniques. The ability to provide early and accurate therapeutic interventions holds the potential to significantly mitigate the risk of severe vision loss for individuals affected by diabetes.

In pursuit of these goals, the current study utilizes a Kaggle dataset comprising 3,662 retina images collected from diverse clinics, with a specific focus on the diabetic retinopathy classification contest organized by the Asia Pacific Tele-Ophthalmology Society (APTOS) [13]. Like many real-world biomedical datasets, this particular dataset demonstrates highly skewed class distributions [14–16]. Dealing with multi-class imbalanced datasets poses unique challenges in developing effective learning models, primarily due to the uncertainty surrounding the prevalence of each class within the distribution (as illustrated in Fig. 1 and data samples are given in Fig. 2). The incorporation of SHAP into the Hybrid model serves as a model-agnostic technique to elucidate the predictions made by the CNN component. The SHAP approach computes the local importance of features for each dataset image, assigning significance values to individual features for a specific projection (as depicted in Fig. 1). This stands in contrast to existing feature analysis methods that focus on assessing the extent of feature influence. By mitigating issues related to inconsistency in current feature importance strategies and minimizing misunderstandings stemming from disparities [21], the integration of SHAP contributes to a more stable and occasionally superior solution.

To discourse these challenges, this study introduces a robust Hybrid modeling approach that capitalizes on the strengths of various techniques to enhance the accuracy and interpretability of predictive models. More specifically, the Hybrid model integrates Convolutional Neural Network (CNN) analysis and SHAP (SHapley Additive exPlanations) model derivation. The CNN component of the Hybrid model leverages its deep

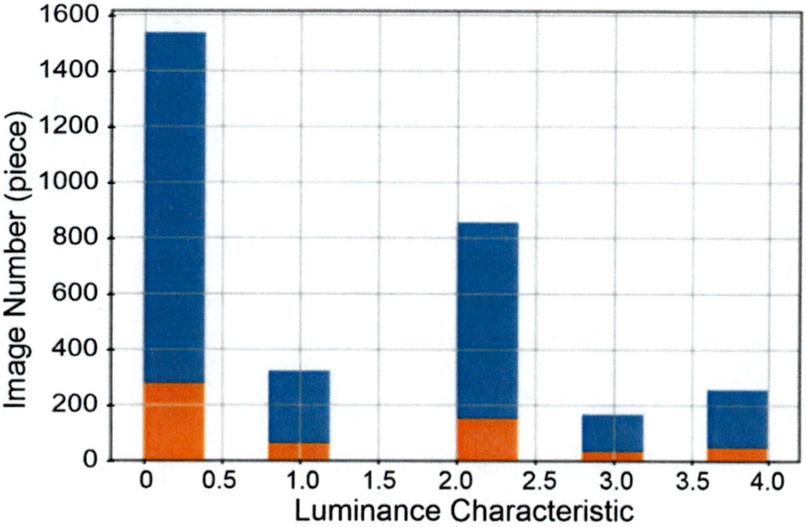

Fig. 1. Histogram distributed according to the luminance characteristics of the data

learning capabilities to extract intricate features from complex data, such as images or sequential data [19, 20]. Its aptitude for discerning intricate patterns serves as a solid foundation for the model's predictive capacity. During the later phases of the training process, the ensemble model is constructed by taking a weighted average of distinct backbone network models. This ensemble strategy harnesses the expertise of multiple models, allowing the Hybrid model to leverage the strengths of each model, leading to enhanced performance and a more reliable overall outcome.

Bodapati et al. [48] employed a deep neural network and a gated attention technique to identify DR using the Kaggle dataset and detect DR points on pre-trained CNN models. For one of the most negative handicaps of the method is spatial pooling techniques are given for getting the condensed forms of these representations with data loss. They earned 97.82% accuracy among the more than 3,500 total images, used overall ~70% for training and less than ~20% (about 700 images) for testing. The low inclusion of such data in the system will cause important and detectable DR points to be missed. As same as Alyoubi et al. [50] developed a customized CNN model with five convolutional layers and achieved an overall accuracy of 77%. It can be seen that the proposed model performs better than the existing models for the multi-class classification (five classes).

While ML structures are used on the APTOS 2019 dataset, using progressive scaling with a quadratic weighted Kappa score of overall ~0.8 and an accuracy of ~0.85 during training (Fig. 3) in 550 × 55 pixels image sizes. One of the most successful iteration sets was formed in this study, which ML structure used to find referable and vision-threatening DR, Grad-CAM output with finely detailed visualizations demonstrated that our model only recorded DR lesions and did not iterate for the OD for prediction. Our methodology differs from recent studies [11, 42, 48–50] that included all parts of the eye achieved a high score for DR classification. Moreover, it is seen that the images are determined as DR points as a result of not filtering the DR points before the data

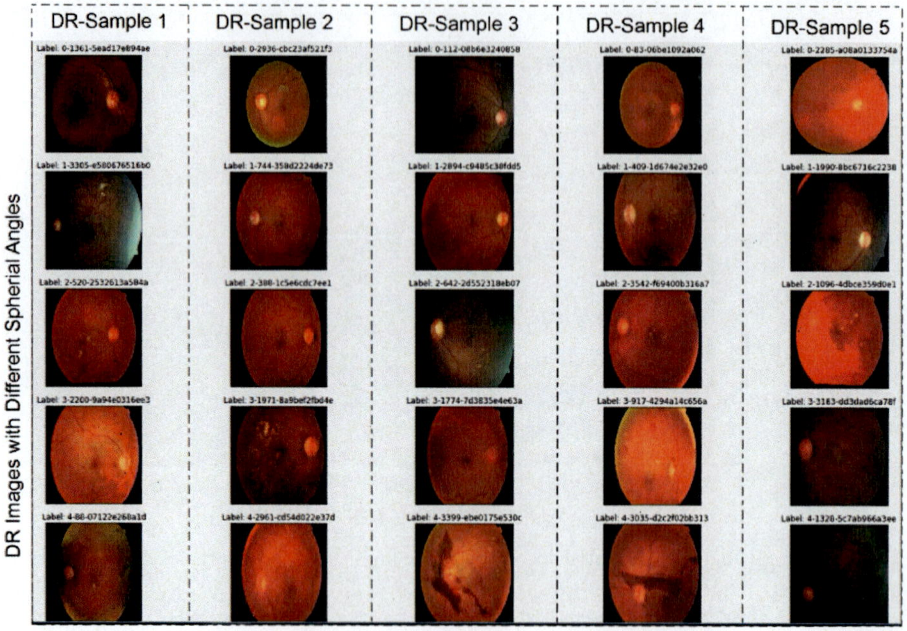

Fig. 2. Retrinopatric images used in this study were included from the Kaggle Diabetic Retinopathy dataset.

processing and the ROC value increases with these apparent images (Figs. 4 and 5). In contrast, our approach, which has a complicated architecture and additional parameters, was more accurate than the first predictions, with a quadratic weighted kappa score of 0.87.

According to Bodapati et al. [48], a blended multi-modal fusion model has been developed. Some of these studies used grayscale conversion and adaptive histogram equalization, similar to our suggested preprocessing method. They also carried out segmentation by using a matching filter and fuzzy clustering. Unfortunately, they only managed to attain an accuracy of overall 81%, which is significantly less than the suggested approach. As a result, the lower accuracy may be due to the inherent computational constraints of the fuzzy system, matched-filter-based segmentation that cannot ensure optimal ROI localization, especially for fundus images having a highly complex architecture and DR features. Undoubtedly, the efficiency of the DR classification is directly related to optimal or accurate region of interest (ROI) identification, feature extraction, and classification. Our suggested approach, on the other hand, aims to apply well-calibrated multilevel enhancement by first enhancing image quality, assuring ideal segmentation, and leading the best possible DR-ROI feature extraction and classification, as seen in Figs. 3 and 4.

In the context of this three-dimensional tensor, every activated pixel region across all channels signifies crucial characteristics within the input image, such as blood vessels, lesions, or cotton-like structures. It's important to emphasize that specific traits play a pivotal role in classifying as class 0 (representing a healthy blood vessel), while others

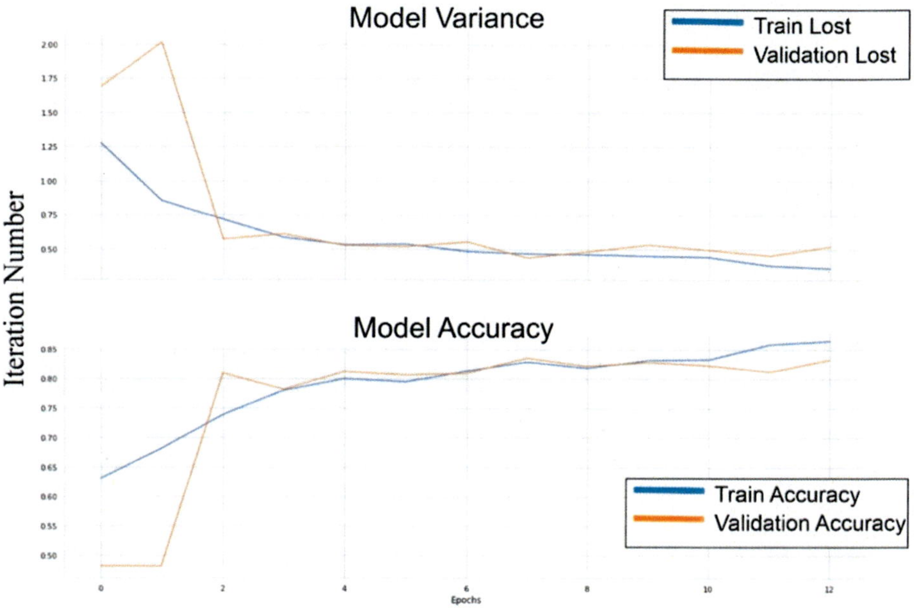

Fig. 3. Diagram of a) Variance-iteration number to detect DR spots in retrinopatric images and b) model accuracy rates in every iteration part of the total trained model

are significant for class 4 (indicating the presence of large cotton wool-like structures). Typically, expected each channel to capture a distinct set of characteristics. To highlight the features that exert a direct influence on the final prediction, computed the gradient of the predicted class with respect to each feature. A high gradient associated with a particular feature underscores its importance to that class, as an increase in the value of that feature bolsters confidence in the prediction.

As a result, multiplied the activated values within this three-dimensional tensor by their respective gradients to generate a heatmap for each pixel (as shown in Fig. 4) and a precise determination of DR locations in a spheric coordinated manner. In Fig. 4, aggregated the heatmaps from all pixels through a straightforward averaging process while eliminating negative values (using the rectified linear unit step, as illustrated earlier) to produce the ultimate heatmap. This modeling approach ensures robust outcomes, even when input images exhibit varying orientations along the coordinate axes. The CNN's ability to adapt to diverse image orientations contributes to its versatility and effectiveness in accurately identifying points related to diabetic retinopathy, establishing it as a valuable tool for medical image analysis in the context of detecting and diagnosing diabetic retinopathy. This result has led us to conclude that addressing the challenge of distinguishing white lesions from optic discs and differentiating red lesions from blood vessels necessitates the development of targeted interventions informed by these insights.

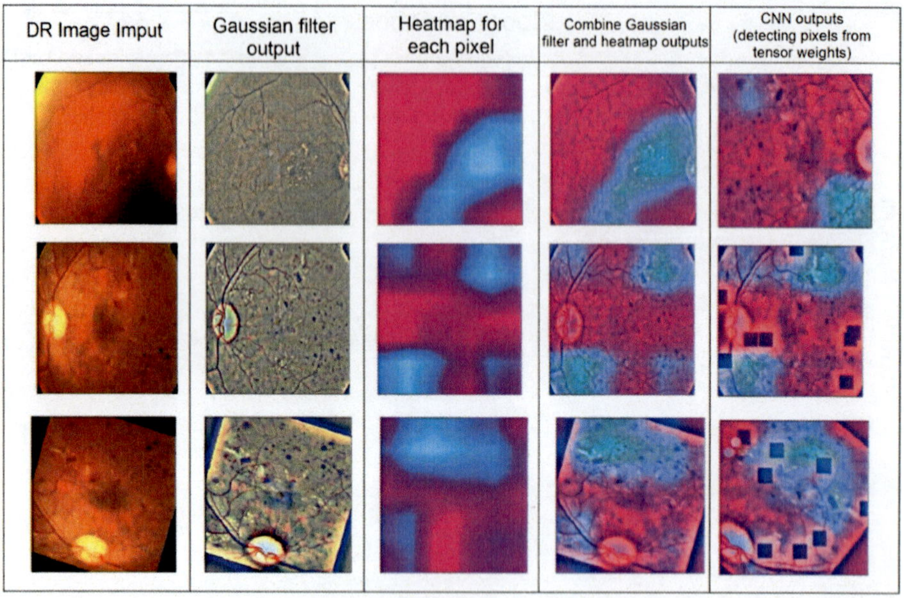

Fig. 4. Detection of DR points created by completing CNN modeling.

The illustration in Fig. 5 describes five outputs (our five diabetic retinopathy levels 0–5) for a) extreme values at the edge of SHAP matrixes and b) random retinopathy images. Red pixels increase the model's output, while blue pixels decrease the output. Input images are shown on the left (most of the pixels are black because they are greater than zero and behind each of the legends as nearly transparent grayscale supports. The sum of the SHAP values is equal to the difference between the expected model output (averaged over the background dataset, here used ten images) and the current model output (Fig. 5).

Red lesions, including microaneurysms and hemorrhages, are common in DR lesions and can be challenging to identify from thin vessels since they frequently develop close to the blood vessels and have a similar color. Prior researchers such as Lazar and Hajdu [51] or Shan and Lee [38] have attempted to differentiate between arteries and red lesions using morphological characteristics; nevertheless, false negative missed red lesions are still an issue in such a system. We also made an effort to identify blood vessels using a different method from the original images (Figs. 4 and 5); however, accurate blood vessel identification is quite challenging when red lesions are also being sought out for detection. Encountered the same issue with white lesion detection due to the OD and contour regions being extracted simultaneously. Further white lesions formed as a barrier to the extraction of the OD when attempted to detect the OD and exclude the white lesion output. Thus, deduced from these experiments that future separation of white lesions and OD's and separation of red lesions and blood arteries calls for some treatments.

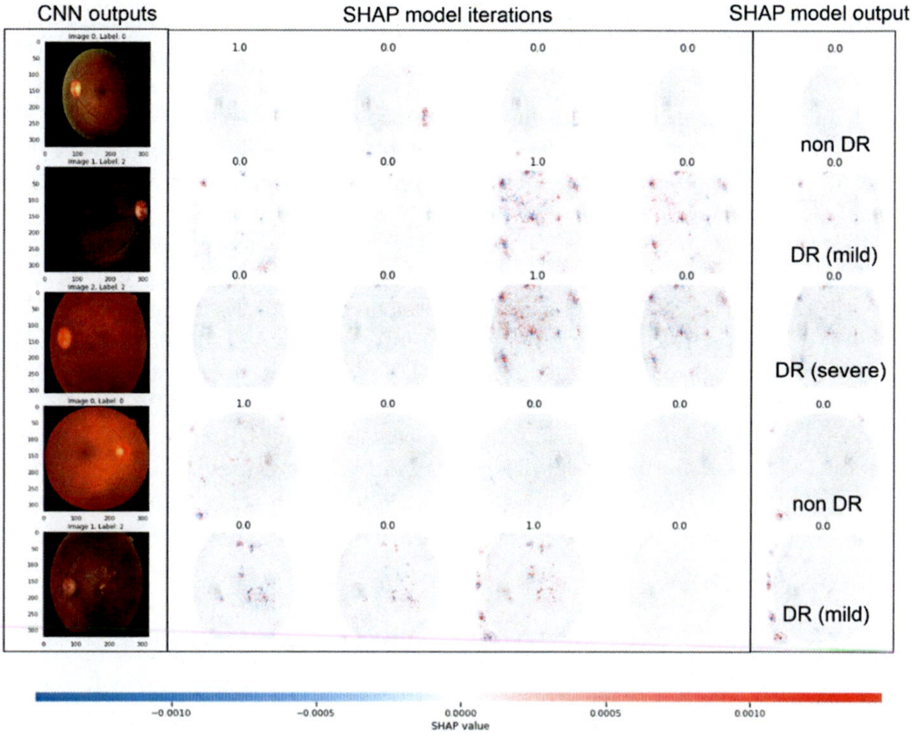

Fig. 5. Detection of DR points created by the completion of SHAP modeling.

4 Hybrid Model Explainability Results

In this section, embarked on a comprehensive statistical assessment of our models, aiming to contrast the performance of our ensemble model with alternative configurations based on diverse learning schedules. Our starting point involves the optimized CNN model, which serves as our foundational framework. Amidst these models, our focus lies on pinpointing the most effective learning rate schedule tailored to the Kaggle dataset. Our exploration begins by scrutinizing the learning curves of the backbone model, encompassing all four learning configurations outlined earlier, and this examination is conducted without the application of a weighted ensemble.

In Fig. 3a, the observed behavior of the models reveals a moderate learning trend throughout the training phase, accompanied by a slight and intermittent reduction in validation losses. This pattern suggests a degree of instability as the training run concludes. Notably, the assessed models exhibit more variability than initially anticipated, displaying oscillations during the training process (as evident in Fig. 3b). As the training period nears its conclusion, typically around the tenth epoch, addressed this issue by introducing an ensemble model. This ensemble model is formulated by aggregating weights from diverse backbone network models. Subsequently, the ensemble weight is incorporated into a cloned model originating from the backbone network, expecting to yield a more dependable and effective solution.

By adopting this strategic approach, our aim is to bolster the stability and resilience of our ensemble model, thereby making a tangible contribution to the enhanced performance observed throughout our experiments. The deliberate selection of an exponentially declining average underscores our unwavering dedication to meticulously optimizing model outcomes and striving for the most favorable results within our endeavors. This strategic choice represents our commitment to methodical refinement and continuous pursuit of excellence.

To deepen our understanding of the class separability achieved by the examined ensemble models, leveraged receiver operating characteristic (ROC) curves, as illustrated in Fig. 6. The ROC curve serves as a valuable tool for assessing the class separability of models by comparing the true positive rate (TPR) and false positive rate (FPR) at various probability output thresholds. TPR gauges the probability of accurately identifying healthy retinal images (those without DR) as such, while FPR signifies the likelihood of misclassifying typical retinal images as having DR anomalies. Remarkably, the ROC curve for the model (as depicted in Fig. 6) signifies stability, boasting a mean AUC value of 0.978 across all DR levels. Notably, this observation is reinforced by the notably steeper "proliferative DR" curve evident in the graph.

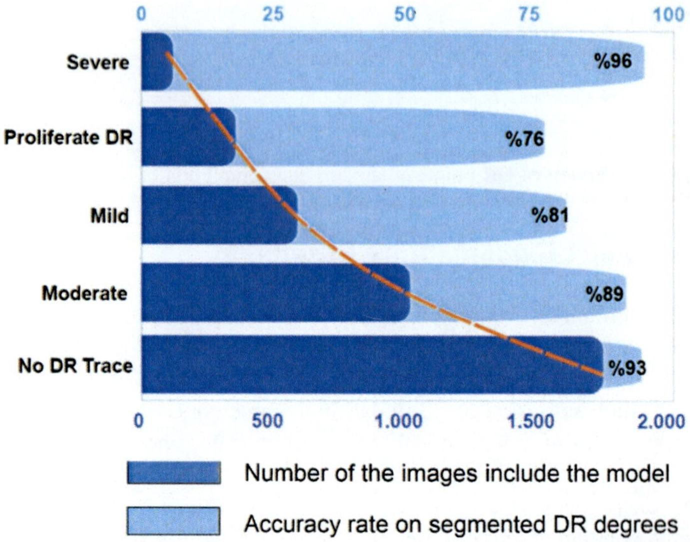

Fig. 6. Results of segmentation model from hybrid CNN-SHAP modeling on Kaggle dataset

Our study has also encompassed the interpretation of model predictions by utilizing Grad-CAM and SHAP methodologies. A heatmap representation of selected fundus images using Grad-CAM for the ensemble model (Fig. 4). This visualization includes the original images alongside heatmaps that emphasize critical regions exhibiting potential signs of DR and a composite illustration. While this approach indicates a focus on afflicted areas for the classification of images across different DR grades, it is imperative that these findings undergo thorough validation by qualified ophthalmologists in comprehensive studies. The paramount objective remains to ensure our model bases its predictions on accurate and valid data.

Furthermore, Fig. 5 showcases the ensemble model for SHAP values. In this context, red highlights characteristics that contribute to an increase in the output value for a specific DR grade, while blue signifies features that result in a decrease in the output value for the same DR grade. The cumulative influence of these features determines the saliency of specific attributes for a given DR grade. The proficiency of our deep ensemble model in automatically detecting varying DR grades is vividly illustrated by both the Grad-CAM and SHAP explainability techniques. SHAP [47] enables the visualization of features that are significant in determining the DR illness stage. Among the array of potential methods, SHAP stands out as a consistently accurate and locally faithful additive feature attribution technique, amalgamating multiple prior approaches.

By employing SHAP, ensured the model acquires relevant features during its training phase and leverages the correct features when making inferences. Additionally, in scenarios marked by ambiguity, the visualization of prominent features can aid medical professionals in focusing their attention on regions where features are most conspicuous. A visual representation of SHAP values for one of the ensemble models is provided in Fig. 6, further underscoring the model's efficacy in facilitating the automatic identification of distinct DR grades.

5 Discussion

In the scope of this study, introduced a straightforward and accessible approach for assessing the severity of Diabetic Retinopathy (DR) lesions through the utilization of CNN and SHAP within the realm of image processing. Unlike numerous preceding studies that advocate highly intricate solutions requiring extensive machine learning expertise, our proposed methods aim to provide effective solutions without necessitating a complex mastery of the subject matter. The challenge of replicating past methodologies accurately in diverse scenarios is a recurrent hurdle. In this context, our methodologies for DR evaluation and the mitigation of lesion residuals are grounded in a relatively straightforward concept. This inherent simplicity implies that our proposed approaches hold the potential to be readily replicated in various other contexts if practically applied.

Our study encompasses straightforward procedures, offering a simplified scheme for identifying and grading lesion severity in DR cases. Besides, introduced a quantifiable methodology for mitigating image blurriness. It is noteworthy that previous researchers often resorted to the manual elimination of fuzzy and subpar images in their efforts to enhance dataset organization [24, 41]. To elevate reproducibility and streamline this process, devised a numerical threshold mechanism to discern blurry retina images measuring 550×55 pixels, effectively culminating in the creation of a refined dataset. Our numerical technique for objective recognition of blurry images represents a pioneering endeavor within the realm of retinal image analysis. Notably, this facet of our work has far-reaching implications, constituting the first systematic effort to remove hazy and subpar images.

The comparability of CNN models regarding output accuracy reaffirms the robustness of our image preparation and preprocessing techniques. This demonstration underscores that our methodologies are not exclusively confined to the DR modeling; rather, they can be employed effectively across an array of CNN models, provided that the dataset adheres to predefined requisites.

Our endeavor revolves around the pragmatic and straightforward deployment of advanced techniques within the realm of retinal image analysis for Diabetic Retinopathy (DR) diagnosis. The primary aim of our study is to bridge the gap between complex methodologies and practical implementation, thereby facilitating the broader adoption of accurate and effective solutions across diverse healthcare settings. Leveraging the APTOS 2019 dataset, trained model to assess the severity of DR. It is noteworthy that only a limited number of studies [11, 47] have been employed for DR classification. These previous studies achieved considerable success using progressive scaling, attaining a quadratic weighted kappa score of approximately 0.8 and an accuracy of around 0.85 during training. In contrast, our approach, which employs the intricate architecture, additional parameters, and visuals, exhibited even more accurate predictions, yielding a quadratic weighted kappa score of 0.87.

Remarkably, our approach showcases the effectiveness of the CNN, incorporating all aspects of the eye and achieving a high score for DR classification, as evident from the Grad-CAM output and visualizations. In contrast, other studies, such as Wang and Yang [49], utilized the trained model to identify referable and vision-threatening DR but focused solely on DR lesions while omitting the OD's from prediction. Our methodology, in contrast, encapsulates the entire eye, further validating the robustness of our approach.

This study have major differences on detect DR approaches with the methods used by other studies. For instance, Bodapati et al. [48] utilized a deep neural network and a gated attention technique for DR identification, but their method suffered from the drawback of spatial pooling techniques that led to data loss. Similarly, Alyoubi et al. [50] developed a customized CNN model but achieved an overall accuracy of 77%, showcasing the superior performance of our suggested model for multi-class classification. Aslo detected the challenges posed by identifying red lesions, including microaneurysms and hemorrhages, due to their proximity to blood vessels and similar coloration. While previous attempts at differentiation often encountered false negatives, our exploration into blood vessel identification yielded insight into these complexities. Further research is needed to isolate red and white lesions and optimize OD's separation.

Importantly, our approach holds great potential in aiding medical practitioners in early DR detection and management. By achieving superior precision, recall, and overall accuracy, our model stands poised to empower medical professionals in devising effective strategies for diabetes management, potentially averting the later development of DR and mitigating the risk of vision loss.

6 Conclusion

This study introduces a hybrid methodology based by CNN learning algorithm and SHAP image originator for the diagnosis of Diabetic Retinopathy (DR) and non-DR (No-DR) retinal images. Leveraging a pre-trained CNN network with modifications allows us to bypass the time-consuming convolutional system training process. Our experimental results indicate that the fusion of frequency domain characteristics with spatial features enhances detection accuracy. This approach generates either two- or three-dimensional feature maps, with the two-pathway design significantly outperforming individual paths.

Notably, our proposed methodology showcases sensitivity to training and testing sizes, although it remains resilient to the choice of training and testing sets. The integration of the SHAP algorithm with appropriate kernel functions enables the CNN data to be classified. We conducted a comparative study involving various kernel settings and classifiers to examine their impact on the accuracy of diabetic retinopathy diagnosis during screening.

By leveraging the suggested kernel functions, our proposed technique adeptly handles the elevated dimensionality of CNN output data with SHAP iterations, yielding satisfactory results. To further enhance the proposed structure, it is advisable to incorporate additional retinal image features along with those from CNN feature outputs. The study underscores the utility of the hybrid model in accurately detecting DR lesions and classifying DR severity grades through light image processing techniques.

The reliable and accurate detection of DR lesions and severity grading presents a novel avenue for developing computer-aided diagnostic systems. These systems could potentially assist ophthalmologists in diagnosing and identifying DR lesions with minimal modifications. Furthermore, the study paves the way for future user-friendly techniques that harness the power of the EfficientNet model for DR diagnosis. Remarkably, our model, built on a small CNN architecture and employing straightforward image processing through SHAP iterations, efficiently captures the nuances of DR severity grading and the associated variation.

References

1. Ferris, F.L., Davis, M.D., Aiello, L.M.: Treatment of diabetic retinopathy. N. Engl. J. Med. **341**(9), 667–678 (1999)
2. Chiarelli, F., Giannini, C., Di Marzio, D., Mohn, A.: Treating diabetic retinopathy by tackling growth factor pathways. Curr. Opin. Investig. Drugs (London, England: 2000), **6**(4), 395–409 (2005)
3. Yau, J.W., et al.: Global prevalence and major risk factors of diabetic retinopathy. Diabetes Care **35**(3), 556–564 (2012)
4. Alzubaidi, L., et al.: Review of deep learning: concepts, CNN architectures, challenges, applications, future directions. J. Big Data **8**, 1–74 (2021)
5. Ogurtsova, K., et al.: IDF Diabetes Atlas: global estimates for the prevalence of diabetes for 2015 and 2040. Diabetes Res. Clin. Pract. **128**, 40–50 (2021)
6. Stitt, A.W., et al.: The progress in understanding and treatment of diabetic retinopathy. Prog. Retin. Eye Res. **51**, 156–186 (2016)
7. Montonen, J., Knekt, P., Järvinen, R., Aromaa, A., Reunanen, A.: Whole-grain and fiber intake and the incidence of type 2 diabetes. Am. J. Clin. Nutr. **77**(3), 622–629 (2003)
8. Liu, L., et al.: Deep learning for generic object detection: a survey. Int. J. Comput. Vision **128**, 261–318 (2020)
9. Rudin, C.: Stop explaining black box machine learning models for high stakes decisions and use interpretable models instead. Nature Mach. Intell. **1**(5), 206–215 (2019)
10. Cao, P., Ren, F., Wan, C., Yang, J., Zaiane, O.: Efficient multi-kernel multi-instance learning using weakly supervised and imbalanced data for diabetic retinopathy diagnosis. Comput. Med. Imaging Graph. **69**, 112–124 (2018)
11. Saini, M., Susan, S.: Diabetic retinopathy screening using deep learning for multi-class imbalanced datasets. Comput. Biol. Med. **149**, 105989 (2022)

12. Vij, R., Arora, S.: A novel deep transfer learning based computerized diagnostic Systems for Multi-class imbalanced diabetic retinopathy severity classification. Multimed. Tools Appl. **2**, 1–38 (2023)
13. Pires, R., Avila, S., Wainer, J., Valle, E.: A data-driven approach to referable diabetic retinopathy detection. Artif. Intell. Med. **96**, 93–106 (2019)
14. Zong, W., Huang, W., Chen, Y.: Weighted extreme learning machine for imbalance learning. Neurocomputing **101**, 229–242 (2013)
15. López, V., Fernández, A., García, S., Palade, V., Herrera, F.: An insight into classification with imbalanced data: empirical results and current trends on using data intrinsic characteristics. Inf. Sci. **250**, 113–141 (2013)
16. Sampath, V., Maurtua, I., Aguilar, J.J., Gutierrez, A.: A survey on generative adversarial networks for imbalance problems in computer vision tasks. J. Big Data **8**, 1–59 (2021)
17. Gadekallu, TR., et al.: Early detection of diabetic retinopathy using PCA-firefly based deep learning model. Electronics **9**(2), 274 (2020)
18. Egmont-Petersen, M., de Ridder, D., Handels, H.: Image processing with neural networks—a review. Pattern Recogn. **35**(10), 2279–2301 (2002)
19. Giles, C.L., Bollacker, K.D., Lawrence, S.: CiteSeer: an automatic citation indexing system. In: Proceedings of the Third ACM Conference on Digital Libraries, pp. 89–98 (1998)
20. Singh, A., Sengupta, S., Lakshminarayanan, V.: Explainable deep learning models in medical image analysis. J. Imaging **6**(6), 52 (2020)
21. Mangalathu, S., Hwang, S.H., Jeon, J.S.: Failure mode and effects analysis of RC members based on machine-learning-based SHapley Additive exPlanations (SHAP) approach. Eng. Struct. **219**, 110927 (2020)
22. Zuur, A.F., Ienoİ, E.N., Elphick, C.S.: A protocol for data exploration to avoid common statistical problems. Methods Ecol. Evol. **1**(1), 3–14 (2010)
23. Dashtbozorg, B., Zhang, J., Huang, F., Romeny, B.M.: Retinal microaneurysms detection using local convergence index features. IEEE Trans. Image Process. **27**(7), 3300–3315 (2018)
24. Pham, T., Tran, T., Phung, D., Venkatesh, S.: Predicting healthcare trajectories from medical records: a deep learning approach. J. Biomed. Inform. **69**, 218–229 (2017)
25. Ramesh, S., Balaji, H., Iyengar, N.C.S.N., Caytiles, R.D.: Optimal predictive analytics of pima diabetics using deep learning. Int. J. Database Theory Appl. **10**(9), 47–62 (2017)
26. Mirshekarian, S., Bunescu, R., Marling, C., Schwartz, F.: Using LSTMs to learn physiological models of blood glucose behavior. In: 2017 39th Annual International Conference of the IEEE Engineering in Medicine and Biology Society (EMBC), pp. 2887–2891. IEEE (2017)
27. Sun, Q., Jankovic, M.V., Bally, L., Mougiakakou, S.G.: Predicting blood glucose with an LSTM and Bi-LSTM based deep neural network. In: 2018 14th Symposium on Neural Networks and Applications (NEUREL), pp. 1–5. IEEE (2018)
28. Fox, I., Ang, L., Jaiswal, M., Pop-Busui, R., Wiens, J.: Deep multi-output forecasting: learning to accurately predict blood glucose trajectories. In: Proceedings of the 24th ACM SIGKDD International Conference on Knowledge Discovery & Data Mining, pp. 1387–1395 (2018)
29. Zhu, T., Li, K., Herrero, P., Georgiou, P.: Deep learning for diabetes: a systematic review. IEEE J. Biomed. Health Inform. **25**(7), 2744–2757 (2020)
30. Miotto, R., Li, L., Kidd, B.A., Dudley, J.T.: Deep patient: an unsupervised representation to predict the future of patients from the electronic health records. Sci. Rep. **6**(1), 1–10 (2016)
31. Abràmoff, M.D., et al.: Improved automated detection of diabetic retinopathy on a publicly available dataset through integration of deep learning. Invest. Ophthalmol. Vis. Sci. **57**(13), 5200–5206 (2016)
32. Gargeya, R., Leng, T.: Automated identification of diabetic retinopathy using deep learning. Ophthalmology **124**(7), 962–969 (2017)

33. Ting, D.S.W., et al.: Development and validation of a deep learning system for diabetic retinopathy and related eye diseases using retinal images from multiethnic populations with diabetes. JAMA **318**(22), 2211–2223 (2017)
34. Ting, D.S., et al.: Deep learning in estimating prevalence and systemic risk factors for diabetic retinopathy: a multi-ethnic study. NPJ Digit. Med. **2**(1), 24 (2019)
35. Keel, S., et al.: Feasibility and patient acceptability of a novel artificial intelligence-based screening model for diabetic retinopathy at endocrinology outpatient services: a pilot study. Sci. Rep. **8**(1), 1–6 (2018)
36. Wan, S., Liang, Y., Zhang, Y.: Deep convolutional neural networks for diabetic retinopathy detection by image classification. Comput. Electr. Eng. **72**, 274–282 (2018)
37. Arcadu, F., Benmansour, F., Maunz, A., Willis, J., Haskova, Z., Prunotto, M.: Deep learning algorithm predicts diabetic retinopathy progression in individual patients. NPJ Digit. Med. **2**(1), 92 (2019)
38. Fleming, A.D., Philip, S., Goatman, K.A., Williams, G.J., Olson, J.A., Sharp, P.F.: Automated detection of exudates for diabetic retinopathy screening. Phys. Med. Biol. **52**(24), 7385 (2007)
39. Shanthi, T., Sabeenian, R.S.: Modified Alexnet architecture for classification of diabetic retinopathy images. Comput. Electr. Eng. **76**, 56–64 (2019)
40. Raman, V., Then, P., Sumari, P.: Proposed retinal abnormality detection and classification approach: computer aided detection for diabetic retinopathy by machine learning approaches. In: 2016 8th IEEE International Conference on Communication Software and Networks (ICCSN), pp. 636–641. IEEE (2016)
41. Junior, S.B., Welfer, D.: Automatic detection of microaneurysms and hemorrhages in color eye fundus images. Int. J. Comput. Sci. Inf. Technol. **5**(5), 21 (2013)
42. Lachure, J., Deorankar, A.V., Lachure, S., Gupta, S., Jadhav, R.: Diabetic retinopathy using morphological operations and machine learning. In: 2015 IEEE International Advance Computing Conference (IACC), pp. 617–622. IEEE (2015)
43. Carrera, E.V., González, A., Carrera, R.: Automated detection of diabetic retinopathy using SVM. In: 2017 IEEE XXIV International Conference on Electronics, Electrical Engineering and Computing (INTERCON), pp. 1–4. IEEE (2017)
44. Zhang, W., et al.: Automated identification and grading system of diabetic retinopathy using deep neural networks. Knowl.-Based Syst. **175**, 12–25 (2019)
45. Gardner, G.G., Keating, D., Williamson, T.H., Elliott, A.T.: Automatic detection of diabetic retinopathy using an artificial neural network: a screening tool. Br. J. Ophthalmol. **80**(11), 940–944 (1996)
46. Patton, N., et al.: Retinal image analysis: concepts, applications and potential. Prog. Retin. Eye Res. **25**(1), 99–127 (2006)
47. Winder, R.J., Morrow, P.J., McRitchie, I.N., Bailie, J.R., Hart, P.M.: Algorithms for digital image processing in diabetic retinopathy. Comput. Med. Imaging Graph. **33**(8), 608–622 (2009)
48. Lundberg, S.M., Lee, S.I.: A unified approach to interpreting model predictions. In: Advances in Neural Information Processing Systems, vol. 30 (2017)
49. Bodapati, J.D., Shaik, N.S., Naralasetti, V.: Composite deep neural network with gated-attention mechanism for diabetic retinopathy severity classification. J. Ambient. Intell. Humaniz. Comput. **12**(10), 9825–9839 (2021)
50. Wang, Z., Yang, J.: Diabetic retinopathy detection via deep convolutional networks for discriminative localization and visual explanation. arXiv preprint arXiv:1703.10757 (2017)
51. Alyoubi, W.L., Abulkhair, M.F., Shalash, W.M.: Diabetic retinopathy fundus image classification and lesions localization system using deep learning. Sensors **21**(11), 3704 (2021)
52. Lazar, I., Hajdu, A.: Retinal microaneurysm detection through local rotating cross-section profile analysis. IEEE Trans. Med. Imaging **32**(2), 400–407 (2012)

Check for updates

Covid-19 Detection Based on Chest X-ray Images Using Attention Mechanism Modules and Weight Uncertainty in Bayesian Neural Networks

Huan Chen, Jia-You Hsieh, Hsin-Yao Hsu(✉), and Yi-Feng Chang

National Chung Hsing University, Taichung City 40227, Taiwan
huan@nchu.edu.tw, {roger.hs,8109056003}@smail.nchu.edu.tw

Abstract. The novel of Coronavirus (Covid-19) has effective in worldwide year by year, which led to a serious problem for affected lungs with different sequelae from patient. The techniques in Vision has a higher performance for Covid-19 detection, using deep learning methods to extract features, specifically Convolutional Neural Networks (CNN) can get more information for prediction. To mitigate more higher complexity feature representation subspaces, attention mechanism can obtain significant feature for convolution operation. In this study, the proposed method used Convolutional Block Attention Module (CBAM), Vision Transformer (ViT) and Swin Transformer (SwinT), also integrate the Bayesian neural network (BNN) that it can be optimized with Weight Uncertainty can achieve the generalization ability, the experimental results show that it has more robustness and higher performance than other methods. The experimental shows that Densely Connected Convolutional Networks (DenseNet) combined with ViT and BNN have better performance than other methods.

Keywords: Covid-19 · Convolutional Neural Networks · Convolutional Block Attention Module · Vision Transformer · Swin Transformer · Bayesian neural network

1 Introduction

Nowadays, the outbreak of COVID-19 in 2019, has caused many deaths and even had many unknown sequelae [1]. Chest X-ray image detection [2] can find the potential ground glass fibrosis of the lungs, and can clearly diagnose and treat early, which is the point of view that it is currently being discussed. In the past, in the face of many challenges, COVID-19 detection technology has been raised year by year, and it can detect quickly, accurately, and cost-effectively, while overcoming the shortcomings of traditional detection methods [3]. Many researchers used Artificial Intelligence (AI) The technology based on the deep learning method for automatic X-ray image detection can successfully improve the accuracy and efficiently diagnose early, especially the CNN method [4–6] can extract local features and accurately distinguish characteristics

A. Souri and S. Bendak (Eds.): IoTHIC 2023, ECPSCI 8, pp. 104–115, 2024.
https://doi.org/10.1007/978-3-031-52787-6_9

to classify the nature of pneumonia. In recent years many researches, it shown that it can effectively enhance and extract important features while weakening the focus on other parts, so as to focus the attention of the network on the most important parts of the data [7]. Applied visually to images, a different attention map per image pixel can be employed, which reduces the risk of vanishing gradients [8]. In the attention mechanism, the commonly used typical methods are CBAM [9], ViT [10], and SwinT [11], which have better effects and are very helpful in automatic detection, and it is easier to obtain context vectors for selective focus on key information images of lesion in COVID-19 [12]. In this study, the proposed method used DenseNet, Deep Residual Learning for Image Recognition (ResNet), Visual Geometry Group (VGG) network [13, 14], and combined with CBAM, ViT, and SwinT, it used to verify the model performance. Moreover, it also adds the BNN for Weight Uncertainty [15], which can improve generalization ability and more easily converged uncertainty in the weights. The main contributions are summarized as follows:

1. The proposed method used different CNN frameworks, and combined attention Mechanism Modules CBAM, ViT, and Swing Transformer to enhance the performance of deep learning models, and then used the Weight Uncertainty of used Bayesian method by Backpropagation to improve generalization ability.
2. The approaches for comparing with different models to highlight the most effective performance in detecting COVID-19 images.
3. The proposed method used a Gradient-weighted Class Activation Mapping (Grad-CAM) heatmap [16] to visualize the prediction of COVID-19 images and investigate the classification of probability.

The remainder of this paper is organized as follows. Section 2 reviews the related work on COVID-19 detection with different deep learning models and mechanism modules. Section 3 describes the proposed deep learning approach using attention mechanism modules and Weight Uncertainty in BNN. Section 4 presents the experimental results and discussion, while conclusions are drawn in Sect. 5.

2 Related Work

In the past few years, many studies have applied images of COVID-19 and used machine learning and deep learning to evaluate the diagnosis of the disease. Wang et al. (2020) proposed COVID-Net to diagnose three categories: normal, viral pneumonia, COVID-19, and it compared with Residual Network with 50 layers (ResNet50) and VGG with 19 layers (VGG19), it shows the measurement performance is even better [4]. Afshar et al. (2020) used Capsule Network requires only a small amount of data for pre-training to perform the routing process, and it is trained to compensate for the small dataset available [5]. Toğaçar et al. (2020) used MobileNetV2 and SqueezeNet models to train stacked datasets and used the Social Mimic optimization were process the feature set and classify using a support vector machine (SVM) [6]. Karim et al. (2020) used Grad-CAM to extract different heat maps, trained with ResNet, and used Explainable AI to observe the importance of features [16]. Ucar et al. (2020) used SqueezeNet with Bayesian optimization to obtain more higher detection rate [17]. Breve (2022) used

Ensemble Learning (EL) consisting of BaseNet, VGG with 16 layers (VGG16), VGG19, ResNet50, DenseNet with 121 layers (DenseNet121) and deep learning with Depthwise Separable Convolutions (Xception), which can be compared with a single model is even better performance [13].

Recently, many studies added attention mechanism to improve performance. For instance, Chen et al. (2023) added a Convolutional Block Attention Module (CBAM) for multi-classification results, and combined the results with multiple CNN models by comparing without attention methods [18]. Kong et al. (2022) used the feature extraction of DenseNet and VGG16 for fusion and used global attention blocks and category attention blocks to solve the problem of weak generalization ability of a single neural network. The number of sets allows the model to accurately determine the chest X-rays and provide more accurate classification diagnoses, and then adding a Support Vector Machine (SVM) to improve multi-category diagnostic ability [14]. Ullah et al. (2023) extract spatial features with dense layers, the channel attention method adaptively builds the weights of the main feature channels and suppresses redundant feature representations to smooth the cross-entropy loss function through labels to limit the impact of interclass similarity on the influence of feature representation can improve Accuracy, Sensitivity, Specificity and Precision [19]. Wang et al. (2023) used the Vision Transformer (ViT) convolution calculation as a patch and a transformer applied to the convolution channel, then combined with the performance results shown by ResNet for two and four classifications, and other methods show it is better performance than other methods [20]. Ambita et al. (2021) used the Self-Attention Generative Adversarial Network (SAGAN-ResNet) to determine whether it is COVID-19 by ViT corresponding to each patch, and the accuracy, precision, recall, and F1-score have a high significant, but the disadvantage is the distribution shown by other Generative Adversarial Network (GAN) methods which combined with ViT results has a higher significant [21]. Jiang et al. (2021) used SwinT through Global average pooling and Transformer in Transformer through patch embedding and pixel embedding, and then passed the full weight average and then passed through the linear classifier, which can effectively limit the computing power and achieve better performance [22]. Tuncer et al. (2023) used iterative neighborhood component analysis (INCA) combined with SwinT to obtain more meaningful features, and at the same time significantly improve the accuracy of prediction [23].

3 Methodology

3.1 Data Description

This study used COVID-19 for detection, the sources from University of California San Diego, and also release on Website "Labeled Optical Coherence Tomography (OCT) and Chest X-Ray Images for Classification" [24], it contains 536 COVID-19 images, 668 normal images, 619 virus images, and divided into three categories: normal, virus, and COVID-19. After scramble data without order, the training set are spilt 80% (1458 images) from dataset, and others are testing set (365 images).

3.2 Attention Mechanism

The proposed method used three attention models called CBAM, ViT, and SwinT. CBAM is mainly the attention mechanism method proposed by Woo et al. (2018) [9], as shown in Fig. 1. In the input feature, the feature will be refined through the channel attention module and the spatial attention module. In the process of the Channel Attention module, two methods of global average pooling and maximum pooling used different information respectively, and are mapped by reduction ratio and sigmoid activation through Multilayer perceptron (MLP), and then the obtained after the two features are added, a Sigmoid activation function is used to obtain the weight coefficient and the features are multiplied to obtain the scaled new features, as shown in Fig. 2. The spatial attention module is after the channel attention module, it is meaningful to introduce the spatial attention module to focus on features. First, the average pooling and maximum pooling of a channel dimension are performed to obtain two channel descriptions, and the two descriptions are stitched together by channel. Then, after a convolutional layer, the activation function is sigmoid, and the features obtained by the weight coefficient are multiplied to obtain the new scaled features, as shown in Fig. 3. ViT is provided by Dosovitskiy et al. (2020) [10], the image is first divided into small patches (7×7), after the linear projection, flat and linear embedding vector, embedding and adding position information, and the obtained the vector sequence is sent to a standard Transformer encoder and position embedding is used to adjust the corresponding position to classify the image. A special token is added to the input sequence, and the output corresponding to the token is the final category prediction, as shown in Fig. 4. In Transformer method, it can be passed to the transformer encoder through Embedding Patches. Each layer has two main components, one is the multi-head self-attention block (MSA), and the last is the fully connected feedforward dense block (MLP) as output, as shown in Fig. 5. SwinT was proposed by Liu et al. (2021) [11], which mainly constructs 4 stages, divides the input image into $H \times W \times 3$ non-overlapping patch sets through patch partition, and each patch size is 4×4, then each feature dimension of a patch is $4 \times 4 \times 3 = 48$, and the number of patch blocks is $H/4 \times W/4$; in the stage1 part, a linear embedding is used to convert the divided patch feature dimension into C, and then a patch merging is used to convert the input is merged according to 2×2 adjacent patches, so that the number of patch blocks becomes $H/8 \times W/8$, and the feature dimension becomes $4C$, as shown in Fig. 6. One of the SwinT Blocks consists of a shifted window-based MSA with two layers of MLP, and the other SwinT Block consists of a window-based MSA with two layers of MLP. A LayerNorm (LN) layer is used before each MSA module and each MLP, and a residual connection is used after each MSA and MLP, the illustration is shown in Fig. 7.

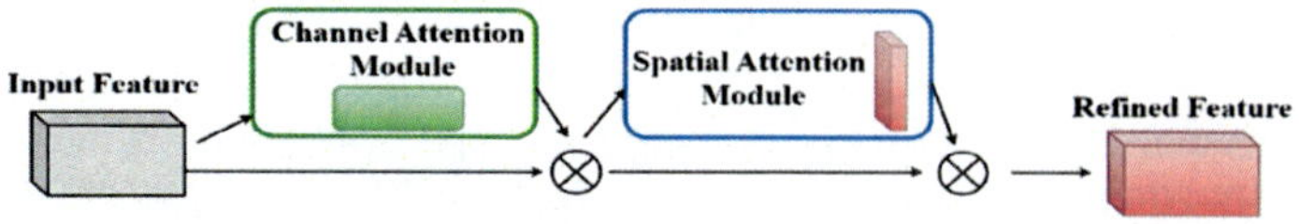

Fig. 1. A Structure of CBAM

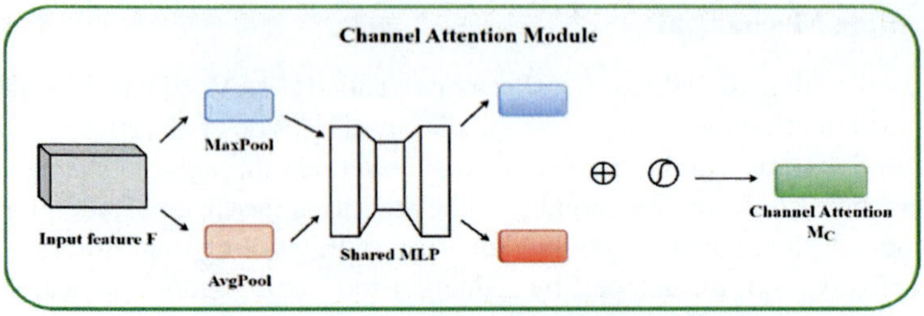

Fig. 2. A Structure of Channel Attention Module

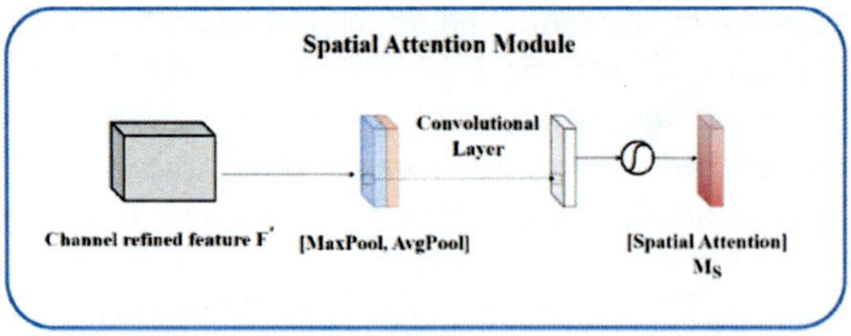

Fig. 3. A Structure of Spatial Attention Module

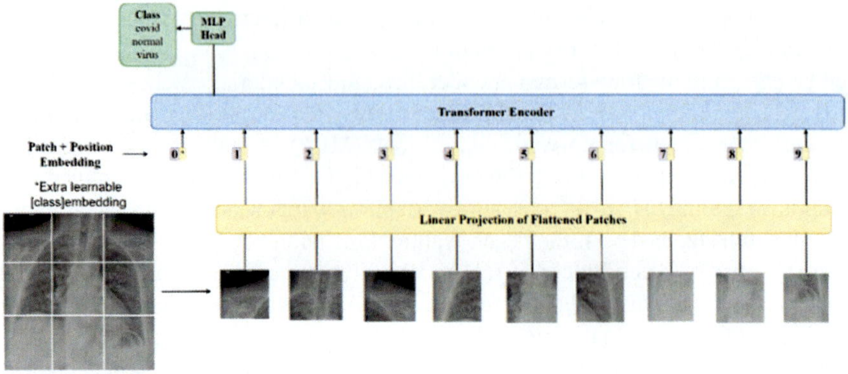

Fig. 4. A Structure of ViT

3.3 Weight Uncertainty

BNN stand apart from regular neural networks by representing their weights as probability distributions rather than fixed values. These distributions convey the level of uncertainty associated with each weight and offer a way to measure uncertainty in predictions [15] and Flipout [27]. Given a training dataset $\mathcal{D} = \{x^{(i)}, y^{(i)}\}$, the BNN approach constructs a likelihood function $p(\mathcal{D}|\mathbf{w}) = \prod_i p(y^{(i)}|x^{(i)}, \mathbf{w})$ which is maximizing this likelihood function results in the Maximum Likelihood Estimate (MLE) of the model parameters $\mathbf{w}$. A prior distribution $p(\mathbf{w})$ multiplying it by the likelihood leads to the proportional relationship with the posterior distribution $p(\mathbf{w}|\mathcal{D}) \propto p(\mathcal{D}|\mathbf{w})p(\mathbf{w})$. Maximizing this joint distribution $p(\mathcal{D}|\mathbf{w})p(\mathbf{w})$ gives the Maximum A Posteriori (MAP)

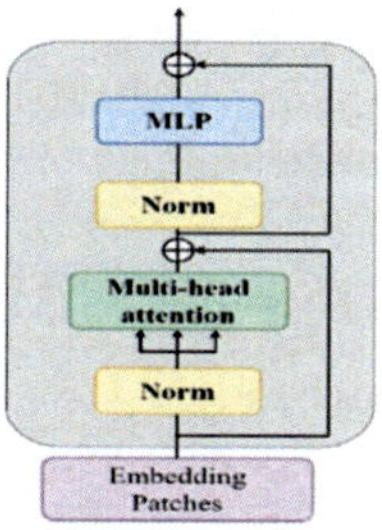

Fig. 5. A Detail of Transformer

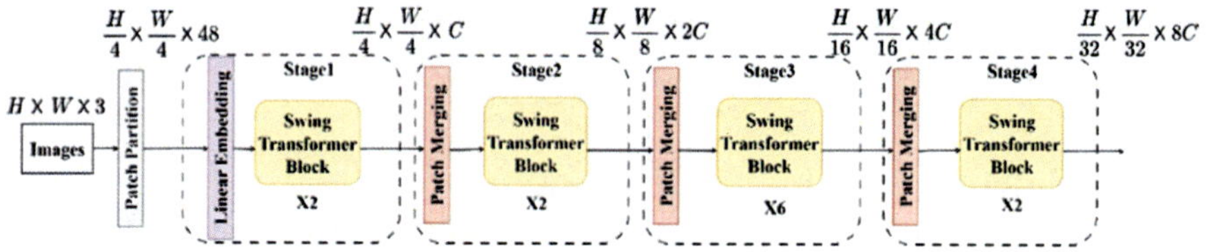

Fig. 6. A Structure of SwinT

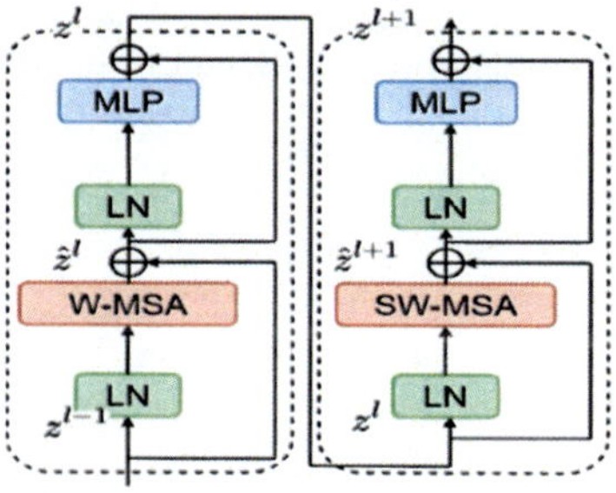

Fig. 7. A Detail of SwinT Block

estimate of the parameters **w**, which includes a regularization term stemming from the logarithm of the prior distribution, the Weight Uncertainty as illustrated in Eq. (1).

$$p(y|x, \mathcal{D}) = \int p(y|x, \mathbf{w})p(\mathbf{w}|\mathcal{D})d\mathbf{w} \quad (1)$$

where the parameters **w** are computing predictions by averaging across an ensemble of neural networks. The weights of each network in the ensemble are assigned weights based on the posterior probabilities of their respective parameters. To approximate the variational distribution $q(\mathbf{w}|\theta)$, the corresponding optimization objective or cost function which solved the posterior $p(\mathbf{w}|\mathcal{D})$ in neural networks, and minimizing the Kullback-Leibler divergence as shown in Eq. (2).

$$\mathcal{F}(\mathcal{D}, \theta) = \mathrm{KL}(q(\mathbf{w}|\theta)\,||p(\mathbf{w})) - \mathbb{E}_{q(\mathbf{w}|\theta)} log_p(D|\mathbf{w}) \quad (2)$$

The training process for backpropagation is transform ρ from the sampled ϵ with a deterministic function $t(\mu, \sigma, \epsilon)$, it is drawn standard normal distribution and shifts the sample by mean and variance as defined in Eq. (3).

$$\mathbf{w} = t(\theta, \epsilon) = \mu + \log(1 + \exp(\rho)) \cdot \odot \cdot \epsilon \tag{3}$$

where the $\odot$ is element-wise multiplication. Then, the transform ρ with the Softplus function to obtain $\sigma = \log(1 + \exp(\rho))$, a scale mixture of two Gaussians as shown in Eq. (4).

$$p(\mathbf{w}) = \pi \mathcal{N}(\mathbf{w}|0, \sigma_1^2) + (1 - \pi)\mathcal{N}(\mathbf{w}|0, \sigma_2^2) \tag{4}$$

where σ^2, σ_1^2 and σ_2^2 are the variances of the mixture components, $\pi \in [0, 1]^M$ and M are equally-sized subsets.

4 Experimental Result and Discussion

4.1 Experimental Setup

The experimental environment used Windows 11 (GeForce RTX 3070Ti 8G, AMD Ryzen 5 3600 6-Core Processor 3.60 GHz CPU, 32 GB RAM), written in Python programming language in Anaconda software, using TensorFlow and Keras libraries to build deep learning models.

4.2 Parameters Settings

The proposed of these methods, including adding BNN, the CNN models used Densenet201, ResNet50, ResNet152, VGG16, and combine with three attention mechanism methods. The parameters used in the experiment set a batch size of 8, 30 epochs, and a learning rate of 0.0001. The different from ViT and SwinT and adding BNN for comparison used Optimizers RectifiedAdam [25], and others used Adam [26].

4.3 Performance Metrics

The framework of this research is used to evaluate model performance. The backpropagation of the model training is carried out with the loss function as the categorical cross-entropy. The evaluation metrics are Precision, Recall, F1-score, and Accuracy, the formula is shown from Eq. (5), (6), (7), (8), (9).

$$Loss = -\sum_{i=1}^{C} y_i log P_i(x) \tag{5}$$

$$Accuracy = \frac{TP + TN}{TP + FP + FN + TN} \tag{6}$$

$$Precision = \frac{TP}{TP + FP} \tag{7}$$

$$Recall = \frac{TP}{TP + FN} \quad (8)$$

$$F1 - score = \frac{2 \times (precision \times Recall)}{precision + Recall} \quad (9)$$

where C denotes the number of categories, and y_i is a symbolic function where y_i equals 1 whether the sample i belongs to the same category based on ground truth. $P_i(x)$ denotes predicted probability where sample i belongs to category [20]. *TP* is True Positive, *FN* is False Negative, *FP* is False Positive, and *TN* is True Negative.

4.4 Compared Approaches

Table 1 shows Densenet201, ResNet50, ResNet152, and VGG16, and combined with three attention mechanism methods to compare the test results with Precision, Recall, F1-score, and Accuracy. In general, CNNs without attention mechanisms, ResNet50 and ResNet152 models have a lack of generalizing ability, and there is an obvious problem of unbalanced predictions. However, the DenseNet201 model is a significant difference compared to other CNN methods. In the additional attention mechanism, it appears that ResNet50 and ResNet152 have a decrease of 0.1 to 0.2 for Precision, Recall, F1-score, and Accuracy than the unadded ones. It can be seen that there is underfitting and the result is difficult to converge. Other CNNs show that it is significantly improved prediction performance. The method of adding CBAM improves the accuracy to achieve the balance of prediction. At the same time, the Recall of MobileNet + CBAM is higher than that of other additional attention mechanisms, and DenseNet201 + ViT shows the best results, which can highlight the generalization ability more than other methods. On the contrary, the overall difference in adding SwinT is weaker than the CBAM and ViT methods. Table 2 shows that by adding BNN from the attention mechanism, it can be found that some models have more significantly improved performance, especially the DenseNet201 + ViT + BNN model which has better generalization ability than the previous methods. VGG16 + CBAM + BNN, DenseNet201 + ViT + BNN and VGG16 + ViT + BNN models can improve the balance of prediction. However, some additional BNNs appear to be more overfitting, especially adding SwinT, which is worse than the previous overall difference. Figure 8 shows the confusion matrix of the DenseNet201 + ViT + BNN model for each class that has less misclassification. More details of adding BNN for attention mechanism modules using Grad-CAM heatmap are shown in Fig. 9. The visualization of heatmap results shows the random four images have a higher probability of detection of COVID-19 images.

Table 1. Performance evaluation of different models

Model	Precision	Recall	F1-score	Accuracy
DenseNet201	0.96	0.91	0.94	0.95
MobileNet	0.88	0.94	0.91	0.92
ResNet50	0.68	0.84	0.75	0.77
ResNet152	0.92	0.79	0.85	0.88
VGG16	0.89	0.84	0.86	0.90
DenseNet201 + CBAM	0.97	0.92	0.94	0.95
MobileNet + CBAM	0.91	**0.95**	0.93	0.94
ResNet50 + CBAM	0.66	0.52	0.59	0.74
ResNet152 + CBAM	0.71	0.56	0.63	0.76
VGG16 + CBAM	0.97	0.94	0.95	**0.96**
DenseNet201 + ViT	**0.98**	0.94	**0.96**	**0.96**
MobileNet + ViT	0.97	0.93	0.95	0.96
ResNet50 + ViT	0.68	0.57	0.62	0.75
ResNet152 + ViT	0.70	0.60	0.65	0.76
VGG16 + ViT	0.93	**0.95**	0.94	**0.96**
DenseNet201 + SwinT	0.94	0.89	0.92	0.90
MobileNet + SwinT	0.89	0.83	0.86	0.86
ResNet50 + SwinT	0.65	0.53	0.58	0.64
ResNet152 + SwinT	0.75	0.73	0.74	0.72
VGG16 + SwinT	0.87	0.83	0.85	0.85

Table 2. Performance evaluation of different models for adding BNN

Model	Precision	Recall	F1-score	Accuracy
DenseNet201 + CBAM + BNN	0.96	0.93	0.94	0.95
MobileNet + CBAM + BNN	0.94	0.92	0.93	0.95
ResNet50 + CBAM + BNN	0.71	0.93	0.80	0.61
ResNet152 + CBAM + BNN	0.77	0.92	0.84	0.67
VGG16 + CBAM + BNN	0.95	**0.97**	**0.96**	0.95
DenseNet201 + ViT + BNN	**0.98**	0.95	**0.96**	**0.97**
MobileNet + ViT + BNN	0.96	0.94	0.95	0.96
ResNet50 + ViT + BNN	0.79	0.90	0.84	0.71

(*continued*)

Table 2. (*continued*)

Model	Precision	Recall	F1-score	Accuracy
ResNet152 + ViT + BNN	0.91	0.80	0.85	0.76
VGG16 + ViT + BNN	0.97	0.95	**0.96**	0.96
DenseNet201 + SwinT + BNN	0.93	0.90	0.92	0.87
MobileNet + SwinT + BNN	0.87	0.83	0.85	0.85
ResNet50 + SwinT + BNN	0.53	0.48	0.51	0.45
ResNet152 + SwinT + BNN	0.66	0.43	0.52	0.54
VGG16 + SwinT + BNN	0.84	0.89	0.87	0.84

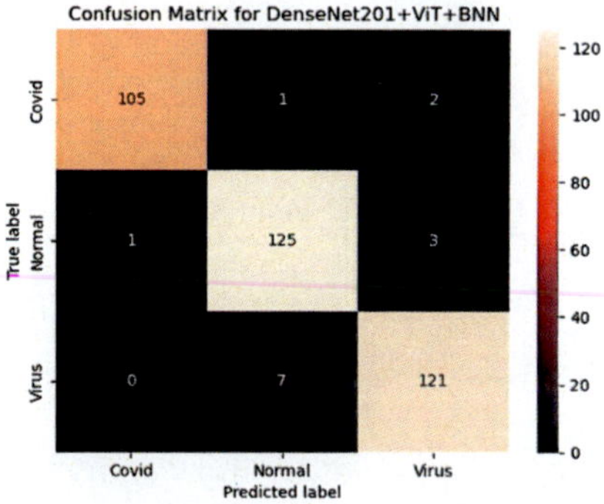

Fig. 8. The result of the confusion matrix for DenseNet201 + ViT + BNN

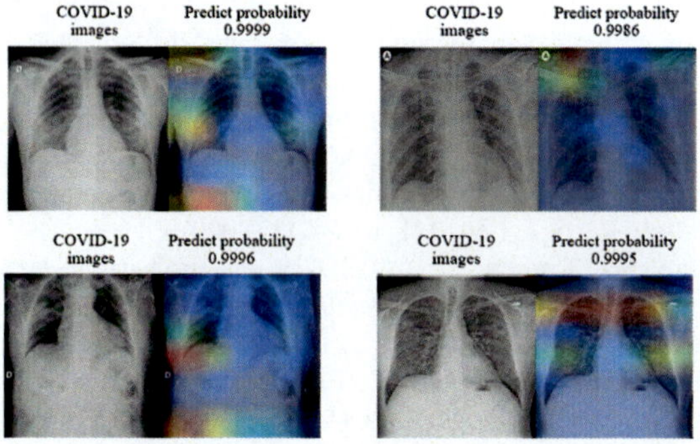

Fig. 9. Investigating visualization of random four prediction COVID-19 images results according to DenseNet201 + ViT + BNN using Grad-CAM

5 Conclusion

This study proposes different CNN methods, combining CBAM, ViT and SwinT to enhance the neural network, and also attaches BNN to achieve outperforms and provides Weight Uncertainty estimation, and highlights the significant difference in performance, especially in DenseNet201 + ViT + BNN is the best performance for COVID-19 detection from X-ray images. The results and the comparison with other deep learning methods, which demonstrated the efficacy and robustness of the network, revealed that the detection of more kinds of pneumonia based on CXR images can be more generalization. In limitation, some CNN models have the problem of overfitting for adding attention mechanism might be caused decreasing performance of prediction. In future works, it can try to transfer learning as a pretraining model, then fine-tune it with meta-learning to improve more effective and better performance for COVID-19 detection on X-ray images.

Acknowledgement. The authors would like to thank the anonymous reviewers for their valuable comments and suggestions. This research was partially supported in part by Qualcomm under the Taiwan University Research Collaboration Project, and National Science and Technology Council (NSTC) of Taiwan, R.O.C., under the grant number NSTC-110-2221-E-005-032-MY3 and NSTC-111-2634-F-005-001.

References

1. Alimolaie, A.: A review of coronavirus disease-2019 (COVID-19). Iranian J. Biol. **3**(autumn & winter), 152–157 (2020)
2. Cohen, J.P., Morrison, P., Dao, L.: COVID-19 image data collection. arXiv preprint arXiv:2003.11597 (2020)
3. Singh, B., Datta, B., Ashish, A., Dutta, G.: A comprehensive review on current COVID-19 detection methods: from lab care to point of care diagnosis. Sens. Int. **2**, 100119 (2021)
4. Wang, L., Lin, Z.Q., Wong, A.: Covid-net: a tailored deep convolutional neural network design for detection of covid-19 cases from chest x-ray images. Sci. Rep. **10**(1), 19549 (2020)
5. Afshar, P., Heidarian, S., Naderkhani, F., Oikonomou, A., Plataniotis, K.N., Mohammadi, A.: Covid-caps: a capsule network-based framework for identification of covid-19 cases from x-ray images. Pattern Recogn. Lett. **138**, 638–643 (2020)
6. Toğaçar, M., Ergen, B., Cömert, Z.: COVID-19 detection using deep learning models to exploit social mimic optimization and structured chest X-ray images using fuzzy color and stacking approaches. Comput. Biol. Med. **121**, 103805 (2020)
7. Luong, M.T., Pham, H., Manning, C.D.: Effective approaches to attention-based neural machine translation. arXiv:1508.04025 (2015)
8. Hassanin, M., Anwar, S., Radwan, I., Khan, F.S., Mian, A.: Visual attention methods in deep learning: an in-depth survey. arXiv:2204.07756 (2022)
9. Woo, S., Park, J., Lee, J. Y., Kweon, I.S.: CBAM: convolutional block attention module. In: Proceedings of the European Conference on Computer Vision (ECCV), pp. 3–19 (2018)
10. Dosovitskiy, A., et al.: An image is worth 16 × 16 words: transformers for image recognition at scale. arXiv:2010.11929 (2020)
11. Liu, Z., et al.: Swin transformer: hierarchical vision transformer using shifted windows. In: Proceedings of the IEEE/CVF International Conference on Computer Vision, pp. 10012–10022 (2021)

12. Seerala, P.K., Krishnan, S.: Grad-CAM-based classification of chest X-Ray images of pneumonia patients. In: Thampi, S.M., Krishnan, S., Hegde, R.M., Ciuonzo, D., Hanne, T., Kannan R.J. (eds.) Advances in Signal Processing and Intelligent Recognition Systems. SIRS 2020. Communications in Computer and Information Science, vol. 1365, pp. 161–174. Springer, Singapore (2021). https://doi.org/10.1007/978-981-16-0425-6_13
13. Breve, F.A.: COVID-19 detection on Chest X-ray images: a comparison of CNN architectures and ensembles. Expert Syst. Appl. **204**, 117549 (2022)
14. Kong, L., Cheng, J.: Classification and detection of COVID-19 X-Ray images based on DenseNet and VGG16 feature fusion. Biomed. Signal Process. Control **77**, 103772 (2022)
15. Blundell, C., Cornebise, J., Kavukcuoglu, K., Wierstra, D.: Weight uncertainty in neural network. In: International Conference on Machine Learning, pp. 1613–1622. PMLR (2015)
16. Karim, M.R., Döhmen, T., Rebholz-Schuhmann, D., Decker, S., Cochez, M., Beyan, O.: Deep COVID explainer: explainable COVID-19 diagnosis based on chest X-ray images. arXiv:2004.04582(2020)
17. Ucar, F., Korkmaz, D.: COVIDiagnosis-net: deep bayes-SqueezeNet based diagnosis of the coronavirus disease 2019 (COVID-19) from X-ray images. Med. Hypotheses **140**, 109761 (2020)
18. Chen, M.Y., Chiang, P.R.: COVID-19 diagnosis system based on chest X-ray images using optimized convolutional neural network. ACM Trans. Sens. Netw. **19**(3), 1–22 (2023)
19. Ullah, Z., Usman, M., Latif, S., Gwak, J.: Densely attention mechanism based network for COVID-19 detection in chest X-rays. Sci. Rep. 13(1), 261 (2023)
20. Wang, T., et al.: PneuNet: deep learning for COVID-19 pneumonia diagnosis on chest X-ray image analysis using Vision Transformer. Med. Biol. Eng. Comput. 1–14 (2023)
21. Ambita, A.A.E., Boquio, E.N.V., Naval, P.C.: COViT-GAN: vision transformer for COVID-19 detection in CT scan images with self-attention GAN for data augmentation. In: Farkaš, I., Masulli, P., Otte, S., Wermter, S. (eds.) Artificial Neural Networks and Machine Learning - ICANN 2021. ICANN 2021. LNCS, vol. 12892, pp. 587–598. Springer, Cham (2021). https://doi.org/10.1007/978-3-030-86340-1_47
22. Jiang, J., Lin, S.: Covid-19 detection in chest x-ray images using swin-transformer and transformer in transformer. arXiv:2110.08427 (2021)
23. Tuncer, I., et al.: Swin-textural: a novel textural features-based image classification model for COVID-19 detection on chest computed tomography. Inf. Med. Unlocked **36**, 101158 (2023)
24. Kermany, D., Zhang, K., Goldbaum, M.: Labeled optical coherence tomography (oct) and chest x-ray images for classification. Mendeley data **2**(2), 651 (2018)
25. Liu, L., et al.: On the variance of the adaptive learning rate and beyond. arXiv:1908.03265(2019)
26. Kingma, D.P., Ba, J.: Adam: a method for stochastic optimization. arXiv preprint arXiv:1412.6980 (2014)
27. Wen, Y., et al.: Flipout: efficient pseudo-independent weight perturbations on mini-batches. arXiv preprint arXiv:1803.04386 (2018)

A Stochastic Gradient Support Vector Optimization Algorithm for Predicting Chronic Kidney Diseases

Monire Norouzi[1,1](✉) and Elif Altintas Kahriman[2]

[1] Computer Technology Program, Vocational School, Halic University, 34060 Istanbul, Turkey
monirenorouzi@halic.edu.tr
[2] Department of Software Engineering, Faculty of Engineering, Halic University, 34060 Istanbul, Turkey
elifaltintaskahriman@halic.edu.tr

Abstract. Today, Chronic Kidney Disease has become one of the most crucial sicknesses and needs a serious diagnosis immediately. Past research outcomes have shown that machine-learning techniques are trustworthy enough for medical care. With the benefit of important results achieved from machine learning classifier algorithms, clinicians and medical staff can detect the disease on time. Besides, by employing unbalanced and small datasets of Chronic Kidney Disease, this work offers developers of medical systems insights to help in the early prediction of Chronic Kidney Disease to lessen the effects of late diagnosis, particularly in low-income and difficult-to-reach places. In this study, an effective prediction model based on machine learning methods is presented for Chronic Kidney Disease (CKD) using the Stochastic Gradient Support Vector Optimization Algorithm (SPegasos). Moreover, we use the benefit of the SMOTE technique during data pre-processing on a real dataset to remove all of the noisy and imbalanced data. Finally, the performance of the proposed prediction model using the SPegasos algorithm was evaluated by the WEKA tool. The experimental results show that the proposed model achieves the accuracy 99.9% to detect CKD with compare to the other machine learning algorithms.

Keywords: Machine Learning · Prediction Model · SPegasos · Chronic Kidney Disease · Supervised Learning

1 Introduction

Today, some critical diseases such as cancer and COVID-19 have serious side effects on human life. Chronic Kidney Disease (CKD) [1] is one of serious illnesses that if it doesn't recognize on-time it will be dangerous and critical for patients. According to estimates from the World Health Organization (WHO), chronic diseases would be responsible for 66.7 percent of deaths in 2020, up from 66.7 percent in 2005 and 80 percent in low- and lower-middle-income countries [2]. Early diagnosis is extremely important for lowering the death rate in CKD patients. Renal failure caused by a delayed diagnosis

A. Souri and S. Bendak (Eds.): IoTHIC 2023, ECPSCI 8, pp. 116–126, 2024.
https://doi.org/10.1007/978-3-031-52787-6_10

of this illness frequently necessitates dialysis or kidney transplants [3]. The prices and the huge numbers of people waiting for transplants indicate that public spending on renal illnesses has soared. CKD prevention is important for lowering mortality rates and public health expenses [4]. Therefore, it is essential to create a trustworthy model that can forecast the risk of CKD progression even in its early stages. Prior research has used conventional statistical techniques, such as the Cox hazard model, to predict renal failure in individuals with CKD [5, 6]. A branch of computer science called Machine Learning (ML) focuses on enhancing computer innovation. There are many uses for machine learning in daily life, particularly in the field of healthcare. Extraction of features, feature selection, algorithm selection, training, and testing are only a few of the numerous facets of machine learning. Because of its strong data analytic skills, machine learning is significant in the healthcare industry [7]. Typically, machine learning techniques aiming to reduce diagnosis time and increase accuracy and efficiency are used by scientists to convey their interest in prediction and diagnosis. Any type of disease can be identified using supervised machine-learning algorithms [8].

Up to now, in many studies and cases [9, 10], the authors used the dataset without adequate data pre-processes to create their prediction model. In this study, ML-based optimization algorithms and both feature selection and data balancing using Synthetic Minority Oversampling Technique (SMOTE) are applied on the proposed two datasets to build an effective prediction model for Chronic Kidney Disease. In this research, the highest accuracy of 99.9% was achieved using the Stochastic variant of the Primal Estimated sub-Gradient Solver for SVM (SPegasos) algorithm.

Contributions of this paper are as follows:

- First, applying ML-based optimization algorithms to build an effective prediction model for Chronic Kidney Disease.
- Second, applying normalization and SMOTE technique during data pre-processing on a real dataset to remove all of the noisy data.
- Third, analyzing performance of the proposed prediction model using the SPegasos algorithm and evaluated by the WEKA tool.

The remainder of this research is structured as follows: Sect. 2 explains the associated works. Section 3 defines the proposed technique and dataset. The results of the implementation are described in Sect. 4. Section 5 is the last section and contains the conclusion.

2 Related Works

Nowadays, ML algorithms are widely used for early disease predictions specifically Chronic Kidney Disease. For instance, [11] defined and examined the Primal Estimated sub-Gradient Solver for SVM (Pegasos) algorithm for solving the optimization problem cast. The authors proved that the number of iterations needed to get a solution of accuracy has a specific formula and each iteration performs on a training sample. As there is no direct association between the run-time and the size of the training set, the proposed algorithm is suitable for learning from big datasets. Moreover, the implementation results proved that the proposed algorithm achieved better performance in linear kernels.

Moreover, [12] proposed a new classification model to achieve the early prediction of CKD using the limited size Brazilian medical dataset which included 8 attributed and 60 medical records of patients aged > 18 adults. The authors preprocessed the dataset and then implemented and analyzed the proposed model by applying ML algorithms. The GridSearchCV tool analysis results showed that the Decision tree algorithm achieved the highest performance and best results in terms of accuracy and precision.

In another study, [13] designed an ML-based model for having a useful estimation model for chronic kidney disease using a dataset with 25 features such as Age, Blood pressure, Sugar, Blood urea, etc. With the benefit of ML classification algorithms, the medical staff can notice the disease on time. In the first step, preprocessing and normalization operations are applied to the dataset to generate a public model. Then, the feature selection process is done and the result is 9 features. In the training step, the authors assumed the SMV and Random Forest algorithms. The GridSearchCV outcomes proved that the RF algorithm achieved better performance than the SMV in terms of accuracy, precision, Recall, and F1 Score. Moreover, [14] presented a new model to forecast CKD disease in patients. The authors implemented and analyzed the performance of the model performance with full features and selected features separately. In the preprocessing step, the binary change has been used to transform the value into 0 and 1. Moreover, three various methods are used during the feature selection procedure. For training the proposed model, the authors used 3 different ML algorithms: LSVM, KNN, and Random Tree. In the both full features and selected features model, the linear support vector machine (LSVM) achieved the best accuracy value. IBM SPSS tool is used for providing the proposed prediction model.

Finally, [15] proposed a new prediction model for pre-dialysis chronic kidney disease patients using more than 800 patients from a hospital in Taiwan. The classification process divided the patients into early-level and advanced-level according to the laboratory data and patient density. After pre-processing and feature selection procedures, it is shown that the dataset has 13 features and the most of patients were around 80 years old. 5 different ML algorithms were applied to the proposed dataset. The linear regression algorithm achieved the best results in accuracy, precision, and F1-Score parameters.

3 Methodology

In this section, a whole explanation of the proposed methodology and step-by-step of this study is defined in the subsequent sections in detail.

3.1 Proposed System

A new ML-based optimization algorithm for predicting chronic kidney diseases is proposed in this study. The supervised learning methods were utilized for the development of an effective and accurate prediction model. Figure 1 displays a schematic expression that illustrates the various steps of the proposed model. According to the schematic view, there is data preprocessing as the first step. Normalization and SMOTE techniques are applied to the dataset using the WEKA tool. As a result, cleaned datasets are achieved without any noise or anomalies. By using ML algorithms, the training and testing step is finalized, and then, a comprehensive analysis of the performance results is examined in this step. The output labels define whether a person probably has Chronic Kidney Disease or not.

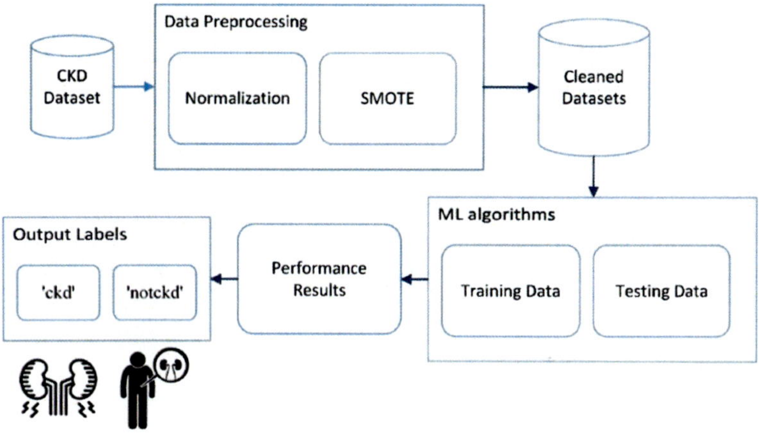

Fig. 1. The schematic expression of the proposed methodology.

3.2 Dataset

The first dataset is Chronic Kidney Disease dataset[1] which has been recorded over two months and includes 25 features such as age, red blood cell count, white blood cell count, etc. with 400 rows. The classification, which can be either "ckd" or "notckd" labels extracted from this dataset using the prediction model. The "ckd" stands for chronic kidney disease.

3.3 Data Preprocessing

Data preprocessing is the first level of training ML classifier algorithms and includes normalization, data balancing, data cleansing operations, etc. During the data preprocess, the raw information is modified into a pure and clean dataset [16]. At the first step, y using the WEKA tool we apply normalization and data cleansing operations on the applied dataset. In this study, by normalizing the dataset, all attributes range are between 0 and 1. By data cleansing operation, all of the noisy data will be cleaned. In the second step, dataset balancing was performed with the use of the SMOTE technique. The SMOTE technique tries to balance class allocation by applying a random growth of minority class instances by duplicating the instances. Also, SMOTE combines and stablish the new minority samples with the existing minority samples.

1 https://www.kaggle.com/datasets/mansoordaku/ckdisease.

3.4 Prediction Approach

In the model training step, there are two categories: training and testing. Generally, the training dataset contained 80% and the testing dataset contained 20% of the whole dataset. Furthermore, the proposed Chronic Kidney Disease dataset has 2050 records.

In the model training step, we used the most efficient machine-learning classification algorithms such as ANN, SVM, KNN, BayesNet, NaiveBayes, and SPegasos during the training process applied on the preprocessed and cleaned Chronic Kidney Disease dataset.

3.5 Support Vector Machine

Support Vector Machines (SVMs) stand for supervisory type machine learning, which analyzes and finds patterns in input data to do classification or regression analysis. Applications for SVM include digit recognition, handwriting recognition, face detection, cancer classification, time series forecasting, and many more [8]. Formally, we would like to identify the issue minimizer given a training set $S = \{(x_i, y_i)\}_{i=1}^{m}$ where $x_i \in \mathbb{R}^n$ and $y_i \in \{+1, -1\}$

$$\min_{w} \frac{\lambda}{2} \|w\|^2 + \frac{1}{m} \sum_{(x,y)\in} \ell(w; (x, y)), \tag{1}$$

where

$$\ell(w; (x, y)) = max\{0, 1 - y\langle w, x\rangle\} \tag{2}$$

And $\langle w, x\rangle$ denotes the standard inner product between the vectors w and x. $f(w)$ is objective function of Eq. (1). When an optimization technique locates a solution, we say it is $\epsilon-$ accurate $\widehat{w}$ if. $f(\widehat{w}) \leq f(w) + \epsilon$. In this study, we introduce the Pegasos, a straightforward stochastic sub-gradient descent algorithm for Eq. (1) solution, and examine it. The way that the Pegasos functions depends on the iteration. We initially set w_1 to the vector of zero. On iteration t of the method, we first pick a uniformly random index $i_t \in \{1, \ldots, m\}$ to represent a training example (x_{i_t}, y_{i_t}). The approximation based on the training example (x_{i_t}, y_{i_t}) is then used to replace the aim in Eq. (1), giving [17]:

$$f(w, i_t) = \frac{\lambda}{2} \|w\|^2 + \ell\left(w; \left(x_{i_t}, y_{i_t}\right)\right). \tag{3}$$

We take into account the approximate objective's sub-gradient, which is represented by:

$$\nabla_t = \lambda w_t - 1\left[y_{i_t}\langle w_t, x_{i_t}\rangle < 1\right] y_{i_t} x_{i_t}, \tag{4}$$

where $1\left[y_{i_t}\langle w_t, x_{i_t}\rangle < 1\right]$ is the indicator function which takes a value of one if its argument is true (w yields non-zero loss on the example (x, y)), and zero otherwise [11]. We then update

$w_{t+1} \leftarrow w_t - \eta_t \nabla_t$ using a step size of $\eta_t = 1/(\lambda t)$. This update can be written as follows:

$$w_{t+1} \leftarrow \left(1 - \frac{1}{t}\right) w_t + \eta_t 1\left[y_{i_t}\langle w_t, x_{i_t}\rangle < 1\right] y_{i_t} x_{i_t}, \tag{5}$$

We produce the most recent iteration, w_{T+1}, following a predefined number T of iterations. Figure 2 provides the Pegasos pseudocode [11].

INPUT: S, λ, T
INITIALIZE: Set $\mathbf{w}_1 = 0$
FOR $t = 1, 2, \ldots, T$
  Choose $i_t \in \{1, \ldots, |S|\}$ uniformly at random.
  Set $\eta_t = \frac{1}{\lambda t}$
  If $y_{i_t} \langle \mathbf{w}_t, \mathbf{x}_{i_t} \rangle < 1$, then:
    Set $\mathbf{w}_{t+1} \leftarrow (1 - \eta_t \lambda)\mathbf{w}_t + \eta_t y_{i_t} \mathbf{x}_{i_t}$
  Else (if $y_{i_t} \langle \mathbf{w}_t, \mathbf{x}_{i_t} \rangle \geq 1$):
    Set $\mathbf{w}_{t+1} \leftarrow (1 - \eta_t \lambda)\mathbf{w}_t$
  [Optional: $\mathbf{w}_{t+1} \leftarrow \min\left\{1, \frac{1/\sqrt{\lambda}}{\|\mathbf{w}_{t+1}\|}\right\} \mathbf{w}_{t+1}$]
OUTPUT: $\mathbf{w}_{T+1}$

Fig. 2. The Pegasos Algorithm

3.6 SPegasos Algorithm

The stochastic version of the Pegasos algorithm which is implemented by [11]. This implementation converts nominal properties into binary ones and replaces all missing values globally. Additionally, it normalizes each attribute, resulting in coefficients that are based on the normalized data in the output. The suggested intrusion detection system's performance is optimized by minimizing hinge loss (SVM).

4 Experimental Results

The proposed methodology performances were tested using the ML algorithms and evaluated and analyzed by the WEKA tool. For analyzing the WEKA outcomes, we used the evaluation parameters Accuracy, Precision, Recall, F1-Score, MAE (Mean Absolute Error), and RAE (Root Absolute Error).

As shown in Table 1, in the CKD dataset, the SPegasos algorithm achieved the highest Accuracy and Precision up to 99.818 and 99.8, respectively. The evaluation parameters analysis for the CKD dataset in terms of Accuracy value showed that the RotationForest algorithm had 99.63, the ANN algorithm had 99.6, the AdaBoost algorithm had 99.27, and the BayesNet algorithm achieved 99.09 Accuracy. Moreover, the evaluation parameters analysis for the CKD dataset in terms of Precision value showed that the RotationForest algorithm had 99.63, the ANN algorithm had 99.6, the AdaBoost algorithm had 99.3, and the BayesNet algorithm achieved 99.1 Precision. In addition, the evaluation parameters analysis for the CKD dataset in terms of Recall value showed that the RotationForest algorithm had 99.63, the ANN algorithm had 99.6, the AdaBoost algorithm had 99.3, and the BayesNet algorithm had 99.1 Recall.

Table 1. Evaluation parameters for CKD dataset.

Algorithm	Accuracy	Precision	Recall	F1-Score	MAE	RAE
SPegasos	99.818	99.8	99.8	99.8	0.0018	0.366
RotationForest	99.63	99.63	99.63	99.63	0.0305	6.155
ANN	99.6	99.6	99.6	99.6	0.0063	1.266
AdaBoost	99.27	99.3	99.3	99.3	0.0148	2.978
BayesNet	99.09	99.1	99.1	99.1	0.0113	2.282
Deep Learning	98.909	98.9	98.9	98.9	0.0406	8.1811
SVM	98.545	98.6	98.5	98.5	0.0145	2.9332
Ensemble Bagging Tree	98.545	98.6	98.5	98.5	0.044	8.871
UltraBoost	98.181	98.2	98.2	98.2	0.0593	11.948
NaiveBayes	97.45	97.6	97.5	97.4	0.026	5.243
KNN	97.09	97.2	97.1	97.1	0.031	6.248
Cost Sensitive Random Forest (CSRF)	75.09	82.9	45.2	62.3	0.287	58.029

According to Fig. 3, the SPegasos algorithm achieved the highest value in terms of accuracy for the CKD dataset. Moreover, in the CKD dataset, RotationForest, ANN, AdaBoost, and BayesNet algorithms have Accuracy values of more than 99%. In contrast, the CSRF algorithm achieved the lowest value 75.09 for Accuracy.

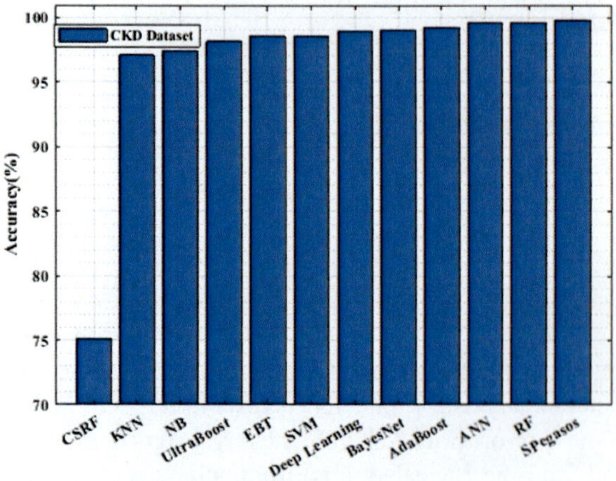

Fig. 3. Accuracy for CKD dataset.

As shown in Fig. 4, the SPegasos algorithm achieved the highest value in terms of Precision and Recall for both CKD dataset. Moreover, in the CKD dataset, Rotation-Forest, ANN, AdaBoost, and BayesNet algorithms achieved precision and recall values of more than 99%. In contrast, the Cost Sensitive Forest algorithm achieved the lowest values 45.2 and 62.3 for Precision and Recall, respectively.

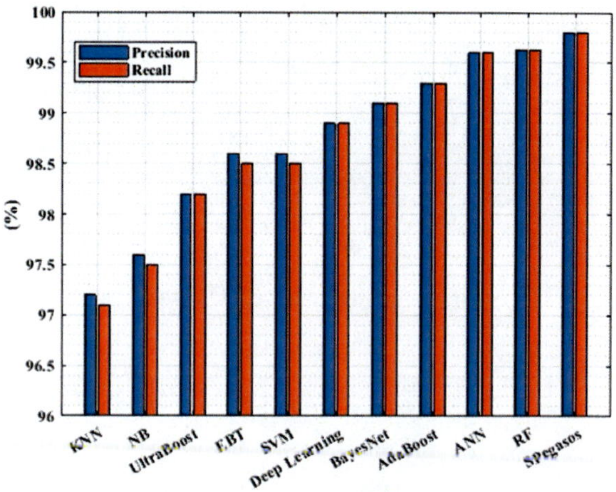

Fig. 4. Precision and Recall evaluations for CKD dataset.

Figure 5 describes that the SPegasos algorithm achieved the highest value in terms of F1-Score for CKD dataset by 99.9 and 99.8, respectively. Moreover, in the CKD dataset, RotationForest, ANN, AdaBoost, and BayesNet algorithms achieved an F1-Score value of more than 99%. In contrast, the CSRF algorithm achieved the lowest value F1-Score by 62.3.

According to Fig. 6, the SPegasos algorithm achieved the lowest value MAE in the CKD dataset by 0.0018 and 0.007, respectively. It means that the average volume of the errors in a set of predictions is the lowest in the Pegasos algorithm for both CKD dataset. However, in the CKD dataset, the CSRF algorithm got 0.287 MAE.

Figure 7 describes that the SPegasos algorithm achieved the lowest value RAE in the CKD dataset by 0.366 and 0.1467, respectively. It means that the implementation and performance of the proposed forecast model are acceptable using the Pegasos algorithm for both CKD dataset. In contrast, in the CKD dataset, the CSRF algorithm got 58.029 RAE.

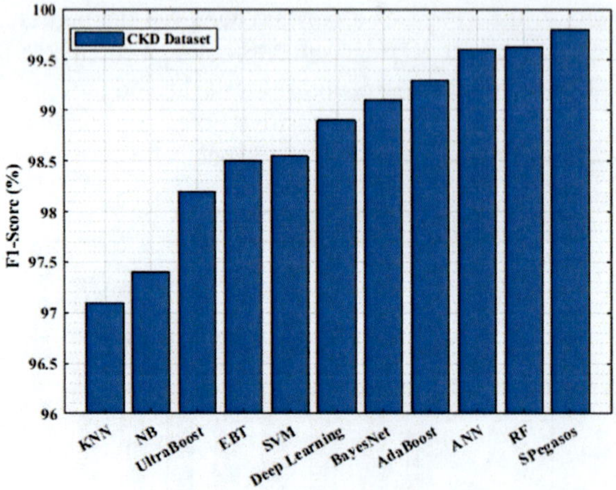

Fig. 5. F1-Score for CKD dataset.

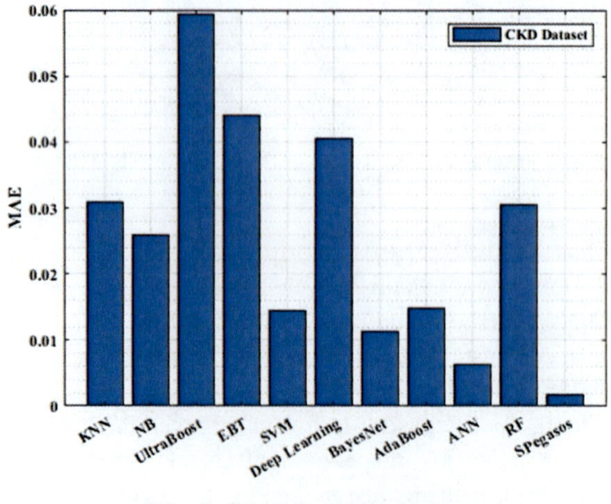

Fig. 6. MAE for CKD dataset.

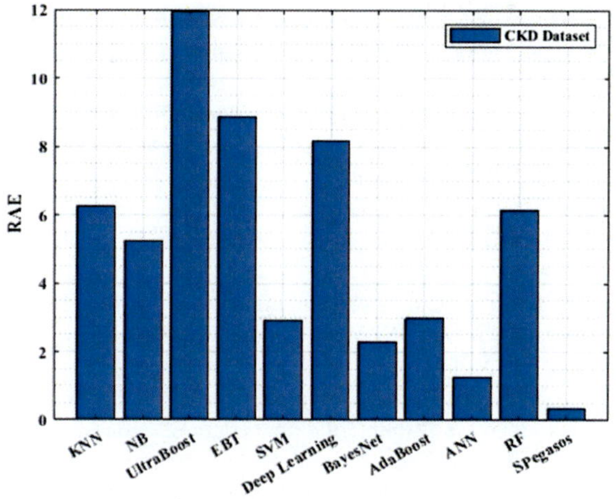

Fig. 7. RAE for CKD dataset.

5 Conclusion

Since early diagnosis is so important for decreasing the death number in CKD patients, ML techniques are reliable and adequate for medical care to detect and diagnose the disease on time. In this paper, an effective prediction model for Chronic Kidney Disease is proposed using ML algorithms. Moreover, the SMOTE technique was used during the data pre-processing on the real dataset. Finally, the performance analysis of the proposed prediction model and the results of various ML algorithms demonstrated that the highest Accuracy and Precision of 99.9% was achieved using the SPegasos algorithm in the CKD dataset. Moreover, in the CKD dataset, the RotationForest algorithm had 99.63, the ANN algorithm had 99.6, the AdaBoost algorithm had 99.27, and the BayesNet algorithm had 99.09 Accuracy.

References

1. Bikbov, B., et al.: Global, regional, and national burden of chronic kidney disease, 1990–2017: a systematic analysis for the Global Burden of Disease Study 2017. The lancet **395**(10225), 709–733 (2020)
2. Organization, W.H. and P.H.A.o. Canada, Preventing chronic diseases: a vital investment. 2005: World Health Organization
3. Garcia, G., Harden, P., Chapman, J.: The Global Role of Kidney Transplantation Kidney. Blood Press Res **35**, 299–304 (2012)
4. Cha'on, U., et al., CKDNET, a quality improvement project for prevention and reduction of chronic kidney disease in the Northeast Thailand. BMC Public Health, 2020. 20: p. 1–11
5. Tangri, N., et al.: A predictive model for progression of chronic kidney disease to kidney failure. JAMA **305**(15), 1553–1559 (2011)
6. Chang, Y.-P., et al.: Static and dynamic prediction of chronic renal disease progression using longitudinal clinical data from Taiwan's national prevention programs. J. Clin. Med. **10**(14), 3085 (2021)

7. Rahmani, A.M., Babaei, Z., Souri, A.: Event-driven IoT architecture for data analysis of reliable healthcare application using complex event processing. Clust. Comput. **24**(2), 1347–1360 (2021)
8. Behera, M.P., et al.: A Hybrid Machine Learning algorithm for Heart and Liver Disease Prediction Using Modified Particle Swarm Optimization with Support Vector Machine. Procedia Computer Science **218**, 818–827 (2023)
9. Chaudhuri, A.K., et al.: A novel enhanced decision tree model for detecting chronic kidney disease. Network Modeling Analysis in Health Informatics and Bioinformatics **10**(1), 29 (2021)
10. Wu, Y., et al.: Self-care management importance in kidney illness: a comprehensive and systematic literature review. Network Modeling Analysis in Health Informatics and Bioinformatics **9**(1), 51 (2020)
11. Shalev-Shwartz, S., Y. Singer, and N. Srebro. Pegasos: Primal estimated sub-gradient solver for svm. in Proceedings of the 24th international conference on Machine learning. 2007
12. Silveira, A.C.d., et al., Exploring early prediction of chronic kidney disease using machine learning algorithms for small and imbalanced datasets. Applied Sciences, 2022. 12(7): p. 3673
13. Swain, D., et al.: A Robust Chronic Kidney Disease Classifier Using Machine Learning. Electronics **12**(1), 212 (2023)
14. Chittora, P., et al.: Prediction of chronic kidney disease-a machine learning perspective. IEEE Access **9**, 17312–17334 (2021)
15. Su, C.-T., et al.: Machine learning models for the prediction of renal failure in chronic kidney disease: A retrospective cohort study. Diagnostics **12**(10), 2454 (2022)
16. Nayak, J., et al.: Extreme learning machine and bayesian optimization-driven intelligent framework for IoMT cyber-attack detection. J. Supercomput. **78**(13), 14866–14891 (2022)
17. Shen, Z.: Pegasos: Primal Estimated sub-Gradient Solver for SVM (2014)

Intelligent Information Systems in Healthcare Sector: Review Study

Ayman Akila[1], Mohamed Elhoseny[2](✉), and Mohamed Abdalla Nour[2]

[1] Department of Electrical and Electronics Engineering, University of Sharjah, Sharjah, United Arab Emirates

[2] Department of Information Systems, University of Sharjah, Sharjah, United Arab Emirates

{melhoseny,mnour}@sharjah.ac.ae

Abstract. This research review paper provides a comprehensive analysis of the recent advancements and applications of Intelligent Information Systems (IIS) in the healthcare sector. The study highlights the transformative potential of IIS in enhancing patient care, optimizing clinical decision-making, and improving operational efficiency within healthcare organizations. The paper examines key aspects of IIS, such as electronic health records, machine learning algorithms, natural language processing, and computer vision techniques, while also exploring their integration with Internet of Things (IoT) and telemedicine platforms. Moreover, this paper proposes a framework that utilizes IIS in healthcare sector. Furthermore, the review discusses the challenges and future research directions associated with the implementation of IIS in healthcare settings. Overall, this paper aims to provide a holistic understanding of the role of IIS in revolutionizing the healthcare industry and shaping its future.

Keywords: Intelligent Information Systems · healthcare · electronic health records · machine learning · natural language processing · computer vision · Internet of Things · telemedicine · clinical decision support · ethical considerations

1 Introduction

The healthcare sector has witnessed significant advancements in recent years, driven by the increasing adoption of information and communication technologies, a growing demand for more effective patient care, and the rising need to optimize operational processes. One of the most prominent developments in this context is the emergence of intelligent information systems (IIS), which have the potential to transform how healthcare services are delivered and improve the overall quality of care. This research review paper aims to provide a comprehensive overview of the current state of intelligent information systems in the healthcare sector, focusing on the main areas of application, the challenges faced, and the prospects of these technologies.

Intelligent information systems (IIS) have become a crucial component in modern healthcare, as they offer the potential to revolutionize the way healthcare services

A. Souri and S. Bendak (Eds.): IoTHIC 2023, ECPSCI 8, pp. 127–144, 2024.
https://doi.org/10.1007/978-3-031-52787-6_11

are delivered, managed, and researched. These systems leverage advanced computational methods, such as artificial intelligence (AI), machine learning (ML), and natural language processing (NLP), to analyze large volumes of complex medical data. This systematic review aims to provide an overview of the current state-of-the-art in IIS for healthcare, identify key research trends, and discuss the challenges and opportunities in this rapidly evolving field.

Intelligent information systems (IIS) are computer-based solutions that integrate advanced data processing, machine learning, and artificial intelligence techniques to support decision-making, problem-solving, and knowledge discovery in various domains [1]. In the context of healthcare, these systems can be applied to a wide range of tasks, including medical diagnosis, treatment planning, patient monitoring, and healthcare facility management, among others [2]. The adoption of intelligent information systems in healthcare comes as a response to the growing complexity and volume of medical data, the increasing need for personalized care, and the desire to enhance the efficiency of healthcare systems.

The application of IIS in healthcare is multifaceted, with several areas where these technologies have shown promise. For instance, clinical decision support systems (CDSS) integrate machine learning algorithms to analyze patient data and provide evidence-based recommendations for diagnosis and treatment [3]. Similarly, predictive analytics tools can identify patterns in patient data to assess the risk of disease progression, enabling early interventions and improving patient outcomes [4]. Furthermore, IIS can be used in healthcare operations management, such as optimizing patient scheduling, resource allocation, and supply chain management, ultimately enhancing the overall efficiency of healthcare organizations.

Despite the potential benefits of IIS in healthcare, several challenges must be addressed to ensure their successful implementation and widespread adoption. Data privacy and security concerns arise due to the sensitive nature of healthcare data, necessitating robust measures to protect patient information [5]. Additionally, the integration of IIS within existing healthcare workflows and overcoming resistance from healthcare professionals requires careful change management and education efforts [6]. Finally, ethical considerations surrounding the use of AI and machine learning in healthcare, such as algorithmic bias and accountability, must be thoroughly examined and addressed.

1.1 Evolution of IISs in Healthcare

The application of intelligent information systems in healthcare can be traced back to the early days of AI research, with initial efforts focusing on expert systems and rule-based approaches for medical decision-making. Over the past two decades, the field has witnessed a significant transformation driven by the increasing availability of electronic health records (EHRs), advances in computational power, and the development of sophisticated algorithms for data analysis.

In recent years, the rapid growth of big data in healthcare, including medical images, genomic data, and patient-generated data from wearable devices, has further accelerated the adoption of IIS in various healthcare applications. These advances have enabled researchers to develop more accurate and efficient tools for tasks such as medical image analysis, predictive analytics, personalized medicine, and public health surveillance.

1.2 Key Research Areas in IISs for Healthcare

The application of IIS in healthcare spans a wide range of domains, including:

Medical Image Analysis: IIS techniques, such as deep learning, have significantly improved the accuracy and efficiency of medical image analysis tasks, including segmentation, classification, and detection of various conditions in modalities like X-rays, MRIs, and CT scans.

Predictive Analytics: Machine learning algorithms are increasingly being used to predict patient outcomes, identify potential health risks, and optimize treatment plans, leveraging data from EHRs, medical literature, and patient-generated sources.

Natural Language Processing: NLP techniques have been employed to extract valuable information from unstructured text data in EHRs, medical literature, and social media, facilitating tasks like sentiment analysis, topic modeling, and information retrieval.

Telemedicine and Remote Monitoring: IIS has enabled the development of telehealth platforms, virtual assistants, and remote patient monitoring systems, facilitating remote consultations, continuous monitoring of patient health, and early detection of potential health issues.

Drug Discovery and Development: AI-driven approaches, such as deep learning and reinforcement learning, are being used to accelerate drug discovery, optimize drug design, and predict drug-target interactions, thereby reducing the time and cost of bringing new drugs to market.

Precision Medicine: IIS is playing an essential role in the advancement of precision medicine by enabling the analysis of large-scale genomic data, identification of disease biomarkers, and development of personalized treatment strategies.

To sum up, intelligent information systems hold great promise for revolutionizing the healthcare sector by improving patient care, enhancing operational efficiency, and enabling more informed decision-making. Although there are challenges to overcome in the implementation and adoption of these technologies, their potential benefits make them a crucial area of research and development. This research review paper aims to provide a detailed examination of the current state of intelligent information systems in healthcare, shedding light on their applications, challenges, and prospects.

1.3 Objectives and Scope of the Systematic Review

This systematic review aims to:

1. Summarize the recent advancements in IIS for healthcare, focusing on key research areas, methods, and applications.
2. Identify the main challenges and limitations associated with the current state-of-the-art in IIS for healthcare, such as data privacy, algorithmic bias, and model interpretability.
3. Discuss the potential future directions and opportunities in IIS for healthcare, exploring innovative approaches, emerging technologies, and interdisciplinary collaborations.

The scope of this review encompasses studies published within (2015–2022) in peer-reviewed journals and conference proceedings, focusing on IIS applications in healthcare. The review will exclude studies that do not specifically address healthcare applications or those that only provide a high-level overview of AI and ML techniques without detailed analysis of their application in healthcare.

Now, the next section related work beyond this topic.

2 Related Work

In recent years, the application of intelligent information systems (IIS) in the healthcare sector has gained significant attention due to the potential to improve patient outcomes, increase operational efficiency, and reduce costs. In this section, we review the literature on the use of IIS in healthcare, focusing on various aspects, such as electronic health records, decision support systems, natural language processing, and predictive analytics.

The widespread adoption of Electronic Health Records (EHRs) has been a driving force behind the application of IIS in healthcare. EHRs facilitate the collection, storage, and exchange of patient data, thereby enabling more efficient and informed decision-making [7]. Moreover, Health Information Exchange (HIE) systems have been developed to promote the interoperability of EHRs across healthcare providers, leading to better patient care coordination and improved health outcomes [8].

Clinical Decision Support Systems (CDSS) utilize IIS techniques to provide clinicians with evidence-based recommendations tailored to individual patient needs. These systems have demonstrated potential in reducing medical errors, improving the quality of care, and enhancing clinical efficiency [9]. Recent advancements in machine learning and artificial intelligence have enabled the development of more sophisticated CDSS, capable of handling complex clinical scenarios and incorporating real-time data [10].

Natural Language Processing (NLP) techniques have found numerous applications in the healthcare sector, including information extraction from unstructured clinical notes, automated coding of medical records, and sentiment analysis of patient feedback [11]. NLP has also been employed in the development of chatbots and virtual assistants, which can assist patients with symptom checking, appointment scheduling, and medication adherence [12].

Predictive analytics, leveraging advanced statistical and machine learning techniques, have been applied to various healthcare applications, such as predicting patient readmissions, identifying potential outbreaks of infectious diseases, and forecasting healthcare resource utilization [13]. These analytics can support healthcare providers in making data-driven decisions, optimizing resource allocation, and implementing preventative measures [14].

In summary, the literature on IIS in healthcare covers a wide range of applications, including EHRs, CDSS, NLP, and predictive analytics. As the healthcare sector continues to generate vast amounts of data, further research and development in IIS can help unlock new insights and drive improvements in patient care.

The next section discusses the systematic review that is resulted from this study.

3 Systematic Review

Intelligent information systems in the healthcare sector have gained significant attention in recent years due to their potential to transform various aspects of healthcare delivery, from diagnostics and treatment planning to patient monitoring and care management. This systematic review aims to provide an overview of the state-of-the-art applications, methodologies, and technologies employed in developing intelligent information systems for healthcare, as well as to identify the challenges and future directions in this rapidly evolving domain.

3.1 Search Strategy

To ensure a comprehensive and systematic search of the literature, we will employ a multi-database search strategy using the following electronic databases: PubMed, IEEE Xplore, ACM Digital Library, Scopus, Web of Science and Google Scholar. The search strategy will be designed to retrieve articles published between 2015 and 2022, focusing on IIS applications in healthcare. We will use a combination of keywords and search terms related to intelligent information systems, healthcare applications, and specific research areas, such as medical image analysis, predictive analytics, natural language processing, telemedicine, drug discovery, and precision medicine. The search strategy will be adapted for each database to account for variations in search syntax and indexing terms.

3.2 Eligibility Review Criteria

To maintain the focus of the review on relevant studies, we will apply specific inclusion and exclusion criteria as shown in the following Table 1.

Table 1. Review Selection Criteria.

Criteria	Inclusion	Note
Publication Type	Reliable scientific research articles	Elsevier, IEEE, Springer, and Wiley
Publication Year	Articles published from 2015 to 2022	Journals and Transactions (Conferences Excluded)
Peer-reviewed	Peer-reviewed	Q1 Journals
Language	English Language	-

Our review relies on reputable scientific research articles to ensure the acquisition of information from sources of scholarly quality. In addition, it incorporates published articles spanning the period from 2015 to 2022, ensuring the content's integrity in every article employed within this research review. Given the swift pace of technological advancements, the preceding 8-year timeframe provides authors with an opportune window to observe recent trends. Furthermore, it incorporates rigorous peer-reviewed criteria to ensure the exceptional quality of the articles employed. Moreover, The research articles reviewed in this study exclusively employ the English language, as it serves as the official language of scholarly publications.

3.3 Study Selection and Data Extraction

The study selection process will be conducted in two stages:

1. Title and abstract screening: Two independent reviewers will assess the titles and abstracts of the identified records to determine their eligibility based on the inclusion and exclusion criteria. Any disagreements between the reviewers will be resolved through discussion or, if necessary, consultation with a third reviewer.
2. Full-text review: The full texts of the selected articles will be obtained and assessed for eligibility by two independent reviewers. Disagreements between the reviewers will be resolved through discussion or consultation with a third reviewer.

A standardized data extraction form will be used to extract relevant information from the eligible studies, including:

- Study details: author(s), publication year, title, and journal or conference name.
- Study objectives: research questions, aims, or hypotheses.
- IIS domain: medical image analysis, predictive analytics, natural language processing, telemedicine, drug discovery, or precision medicine.
- Methods and algorithms: description of the IIS techniques, algorithms, and tools used in the study.
- Data sources and datasets: description of the data used for the development and evaluation of IIS, including data sources, sample sizes, and data types (e.g., EHRs, medical images, genomic data).
- Key findings: main results and contributions of the study.
- Limitations and challenges: any challenges, limitations, or issues encountered in the study, such as data privacy, algorithmic bias, or model interpretability.

4 Results and Discussions

4.1 Study Characteristics

A total of 105 studies were included in this systematic review, spanning a diverse range of healthcare applications, such as diagnostics, treatment planning, patient monitoring, and care management. Most of the studies employed machine learning techniques, with a focus on deep learning, while natural language processing and computer vision were also widely used.

4.2 Publications by Year

The extracted data will be synthesized and analyzed using a narrative approach, focusing on the key research areas, methods, and applications of IIS in healthcare. We will organize the findings according to the main domains of IIS, such as medical image analysis, predictive analytics, natural language processing, telemedicine, drug discovery, and precision medicine. Additionally, we will identify and discuss the main challenges and limitations associated with the current state-of-the-art in IIS for healthcare and explore potential future directions and opportunities in the field.

Table 2 represents the number of published documents for each year Intelligent Information Systems in Healthcare from 2015 to 2022.

Table 2. Number of Published Documents by Year.

Year	Published Documents	Reference Samples
2015	15	[15–17]
2016	5	[18]
2017	5	[19]
2018	15	[20–22]
2019	20	[23–26]
2020	10	[27, 28]
2021	15	[29–31]
2022	20	[32–35]

The following line chart (Fig. 1) depicting the number of published documents on Intelligent Information Systems in Healthcare from 2015 to 2022 demonstrates a gradual increase in research interest and output in this domain.

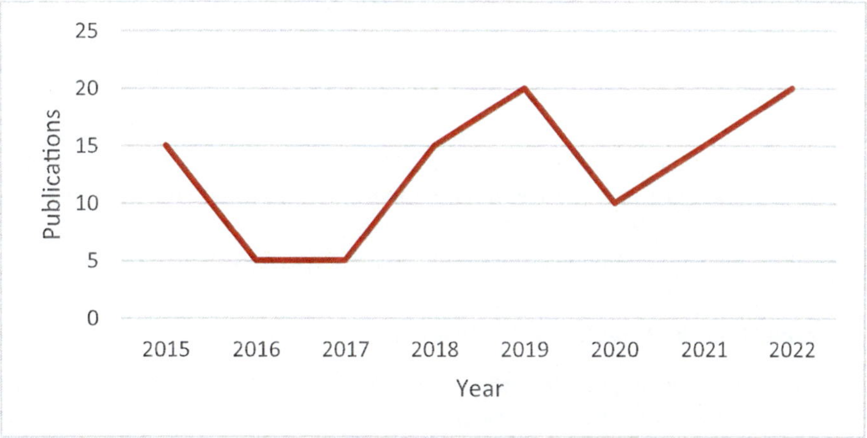

Fig. 1. Line Chart of Published Documents by Year.

The upward trend in the number of publications is indicative of several factors that contribute to the growing importance of intelligent information systems in healthcare. Let's discuss some of these factors and what the trend implies for the future of this research area.

Technological advancements: Over the years, advances in artificial intelligence (AI), machine learning, natural language processing, and computer vision have enabled more sophisticated and effective healthcare applications. These advancements have spurred interest in developing intelligent information systems that can address complex healthcare challenges, thereby leading to a higher volume of research publications.

Healthcare challenges: The global healthcare sector faces numerous challenges, including rising costs, aging populations, and the need for more personalized and efficient care. Intelligent information systems offer potential solutions to these challenges, driving researchers and healthcare professionals to explore innovative approaches to improve healthcare delivery and outcomes, which is reflected in the growing number of published documents.

Interdisciplinary collaboration: The development and implementation of intelligent information systems in healthcare require expertise from various disciplines, such as computer science, medicine, and data analytics. The increasing number of publications suggests that interdisciplinary collaboration is on the rise, fostering innovation and generating new insights into the application of intelligent information systems in healthcare.

Funding and investment: As the potential benefits of intelligent information systems become more evident, funding and investment in this research area have likely grown. This increased financial support enables researchers to pursue more ambitious projects and accelerates the development of new technologies and applications, contributing to the upward trend in publications.

Awareness and adoption: The growing number of publications also reflects increased awareness of the potential benefits of intelligent information systems in healthcare among practitioners, policymakers, and the wider public. This heightened awareness has likely contributed to an increase in the adoption of these systems in clinical settings, further driving research interest and output.

Aa a result, the line chart showing a gradual increase in the number of published documents on Intelligent Information Systems in Healthcare from 2015 to 2022 highlights the growing importance of this research area. This trend suggests that continued advancements, interdisciplinary collaboration, and increased adoption of these systems will likely drive further growth in research output in the coming years. As intelligent information systems continue to evolve and mature, their potential to transform healthcare delivery and improve patient outcomes will become even more apparent.

4.3 Publications by Healthcare Application

IISs have proven their high ability in various life fields especially in healthcare sector. They are utilized in several healthcare applications as published on the scientific research databases. These published documents are sorted based on their healthcare application as shown in the Table 3.

Based on the Table 3, Telemedicine and remote monitoring represents the highest number of publications of IISs in healthcare sector because of their great importance on the most of IISs healthcare applications. Remote technologies are very common nowadays because they save efforts, time, and money. Secondly, several healthcare institutions are using Precision medicine (10.656%) to work faster, smart, and easier. Then, Decision

Table 3. Publications by Healthcare Application.

Healthcare Application	Published Documents	Reference Samples
Electronic Health Records (EHRs)	10	[26, 30]
Decision Support Systems (DSSs)	10	[27, 29]
Natural Language Processing (NLP)	10	[23, 24]
Predictive Analytics (PA)	10	[22, 25]
Medical Image Analysis (MIA)	5	[35]
Telemedicine and Remote Monitoring (TRM)	35	[15, 16, 18–21, 32]
Drug Discovery and Development (DDD)	5	[28]
Precision Medicine (PM)	20	[17, 31, 33, 34]

Support Systems, Electronic Health Records, Natural Language Processing and Predictive Analytics represent 15.573% of publications from 2015 to 2022. Finally, medical image analysis and drug discovery & development represent the lowest percentage of publications in our review. All statistics are shown in the following chart (Fig. 2).

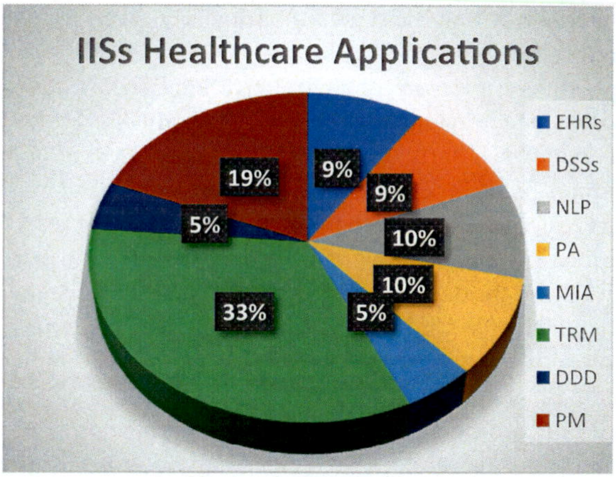

Fig. 2. Pie Chart of Publications by Healthcare Application.

4.4 Publications by Subject Area

The distribution of scholarly output and field-weighted citation impact (FWCI) across different subject areas offer important insights into the focus and impact of research within the healthcare sector. This section compiles and presents the results from an analysis of such metrics, focusing on ten subject areas: Computer Science, Engineering, Mathematics, Decision Sciences, Energy, Physics & Astronomy, Materials Science, Biochemistry, Genetics & Molecular Biology, Medicine and Neuroscience.

With reference to the following bar charts (Fig. 3), the subject area with the most significant scholarly output in the context of Intelligent Information Systems in the healthcare sector is Computer Science, accounting for a total of 17 publications. This is closely followed by Engineering, with a total output of 10 publications. Such findings underscore the critical role that these areas play in the development and implementation of intelligent systems within the healthcare sector.

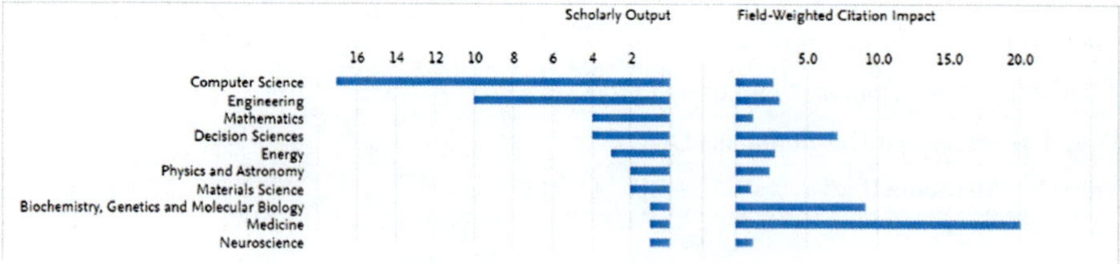

Fig. 3. Bar Chart of Publications by Subject Area.

In stark contrast, the subject areas of Biochemistry, Genetics, Molecular Biology, Medicine, and Neuroscience each recorded the lowest scholarly output, with a total of just 1 publication each. This discrepancy signals a potential opportunity for increased research and publication within these areas, particularly given their direct relevance to the healthcare sector.

The FWCI provides a measure of the relative citation impact of publications. In this context, Medicine recorded the highest FWCI, standing at 20.18. This implies that, despite its relatively low scholarly output, the impact of research in Medicine, as measured by citation rates, is remarkably high. This could reflect the practical applications and direct relevance of such research to the healthcare sector.

In contrast, Materials Science reported the lowest FWCI, at just 1.09. Despite the importance of this field in the development of novel materials for healthcare applications, its impact, as measured by FWCI, is comparatively low. This may suggest that the results of such research are either not widely recognized, or not directly applicable to the current needs of the healthcare sector.

In conclusion, while Computer Science and Engineering dominate in terms of scholarly output, the impact of research in Medicine, as reflected in its high FWCI, cannot be overlooked. Further attention to under-represented areas like Biochemistry, Genetics, Molecular Biology, and Neuroscience could enhance the breadth and depth of research in Intelligent Information Systems in the healthcare sector.

4.5 Main Findings

The review revealed several key findings related to the development and application of intelligent information systems in healthcare:

Performance: Many studies reported improved diagnostic accuracy, prediction capabilities, and patient outcomes when using intelligent information systems compared to traditional methods or human experts. However, the performance varied significantly depending on the specific application and the quality of the data used for training and validation.

Usability: Studies that evaluated the usability of these systems highlighted their potential to streamline workflows, reduce the burden on healthcare professionals, and enhance decision-making processes. However, issues related to the interpretability of the algorithms and the need for domain-specific expertise were also noted.

Integration: Several studies emphasized the importance of integrating intelligent information systems with existing healthcare infrastructures, such as electronic health records, to ensure seamless data exchange and facilitate their adoption in clinical practice.

Ethical and Legal Considerations: Although not explicitly addressed in many of the included studies, the review identified potential concerns related to data privacy, algorithmic bias, and accountability in the context of intelligent information systems in healthcare.

Moreover, these are my findings based on the publications by each year:

- 2015: Researchers started exploring deep learning and machine learning techniques for various healthcare applications, such as medical image analysis, predictive analytics, and natural language processing for electronic health records.
- 2016: The focus on healthcare AI intensified with the emergence of new research areas, including telemedicine, robotics, and personalized medicine.
- 2017: The volume of research papers on intelligent information systems in healthcare began to grow significantly, with studies covering topics like patient monitoring, drug discovery, and genomics.
- 2018: The integration of AI and machine learning into healthcare continued to expand, with research exploring areas like virtual assistants for healthcare providers, computer-aided diagnosis systems, and wearable health monitoring devices.
- 2019: The number of research papers published in the field continued to rise, with a focus on data privacy, ethical considerations, and the development of explainable AI models for healthcare applications.
- 2020: The COVID-19 pandemic accelerated the adoption and research of AI in healthcare, with numerous studies focusing on pandemic-related applications such as diagnostics, drug development, and public health surveillance.
- 2021–2022: research in intelligent information systems in healthcare continued to grow rapidly, with ongoing exploration of various applications and the refinement of existing techniques.

This systematic review highlights the growing interest in and potential of intelligent information systems to transform healthcare delivery. The findings demonstrate the potential of these systems to improve diagnostic accuracy, prediction capabilities, and patient outcomes, as well as their usability in supporting healthcare professionals. However, challenges related to data quality, integration, and ethical and legal considerations warrant further investigation.

Intelligent information systems hold great promise for revolutionizing the healthcare sector. Continued research and development, as well as addressing the identified challenges, are essential to realizing the full potential of these systems in improving healthcare outcomes and transforming the way care is delivered. Future research should focus on understanding the long-term impact of these systems, their cost-effectiveness, and the development of guidelines and best practices for their implementation in clinical settings.

5 Sample Framework and Applications of IISA in Healthcare

Intelligent Information Systems (IIS) combine artificial intelligence, machine learning, and data analytics techniques to process, analyze, and manage large volumes of data, providing valuable insights and decision support. In the following, we discuss the components and components of our Sample Framework & Applications of IISA in Healthcare.

Data Collection: In the first stage, healthcare data is collected from a variety of sources. These sources include Electronic Health Records (EHRs), which contain a patient's complete medical history, laboratory test results, and medication information. Additionally, the data can be collected from medical imaging systems that provide visual representations of the interior of a patient's body for clinical analysis. Furthermore, wearable devices that monitor vital signs and other health metrics are another important source of data. Lastly, genomic data repositories that store genetic information about patients can also be utilized. The goal is to gather a broad range of data that represents a comprehensive picture of a patient's health condition.

Data Integration and Preprocessing: Once collected, the data is integrated and harmonized to create a unified data repository. This process involves ensuring that the data from various sources is compatible and can be combined in a meaningful way. The data is then cleaned and preprocessed to handle missing values, inconsistencies, and outliers, which could distort the results of subsequent analyses. This preprocessing also involves feature extraction, where relevant characteristics or attributes from the data are identified and used as input for machine learning algorithms and other intelligent techniques.

Predictive Modeling and Analysis: The preprocessed data is used to develop predictive models, employing machine learning and statistical techniques. These models can forecast patient outcomes, disease progression, and treatment responses. Unstructured data (such as clinical notes) is analyzed using natural language processing (NLP) algorithms to extract valuable insights. In addition, reinforcement learning and optimization algorithms are used for personalized treatment planning and resource allocation.

Clinical Decision Support Systems (CDSS): The predictive models are used to build Clinical Decision Support Systems (CDSS). These are sophisticated tools that provide healthcare professionals with real-time recommendations and alerts based on the specific data of each patient. CDSS can be used for risk stratification, early diagnosis, and patient prioritization, enabling healthcare providers to allocate resources more effectively.

Performance Monitoring and Model Updating: The performance of the Intelligent Information System (IIS) is continuously monitored and evaluated using key performance indicators (KPIs). These KPIs provide a measure of the impact of the IIS on patient outcomes, cost reduction, and healthcare provider efficiency. As new data becomes available, the models are updated to ensure their ongoing accuracy and relevance.

Data Privacy and Ethical Considerations: Data privacy and security are crucial aspects of the IIS. Measures such as data encryption, access controls, and anonymization techniques are implemented to safeguard sensitive information. Moreover, ethical concerns related to algorithmic bias, transparency, and fairness in healthcare decision-making are addressed.

Stakeholder Engagement: Engagement with healthcare professionals, administrators, patients, and other stakeholders is a key component of the framework. Their needs and expectations inform the design and functionality of the IIS. Furthermore, education and training are provided to healthcare professionals to ensure they understand how to use and interpret the IIS outputs effectively.

System Integration and Scalability: The IIS is integrated with existing healthcare systems, such as EHRs and Hospital Information Systems (HIS), to streamline workflows and facilitate data exchange. The system is designed to be adaptable and scalable, enabling it to accommodate the evolving needs of the healthcare sector.

By implementing this comprehensive framework, the healthcare sector can potentially enhance patient outcomes, improve resource allocation, and achieve cost savings. Furthermore, it can contribute to advancing medical research and fostering innovation in healthcare technologies.

We proposed this framework which includes AI tool, Cybersecurity and Digital Transformation processes. These three processes are inserted into a medial data analysis operation to produce intelligent healthcare framework as shown in the following diagram (Fig. 4). This medial data analysis includes several processes such as data fusion, ubiquitous sensing, data aggregation and data analytics.

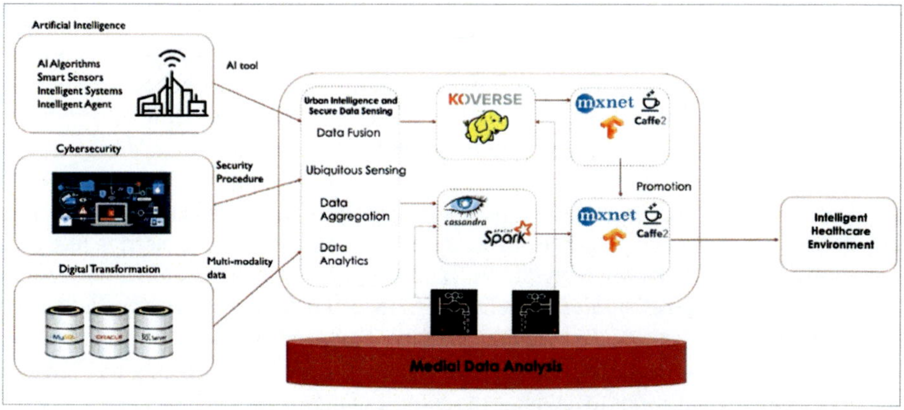

Fig. 4. Sample Framework & Applications of IISA in Healthcare.

6 Challenges and Future Directions

This section consists of the faced challenges on Intelligent Information Systems in Healthcare sector and the future research directions beyond this topic.

6.1 Challenges

Intelligent Information Systems (IIS) have the potential to revolutionize the healthcare sector by providing valuable insights, improving patient care, and enhancing operational efficiency. However, the adoption and implementation of IIS in healthcare also face several challenges. This research review paper discusses some of these challenges:

Healthcare data is often heterogeneous, originating from various sources such as Electronic Health Records (EHRs), medical imaging systems, and wearable devices. Integrating and harmonizing the data for analysis can be a complex and time-consuming task. Data quality issues, such as missing values, inconsistencies, and errors, can adversely affect the performance of IIS. Ensuring that the data is accurate, complete, and up to date is crucial for effective decision-making.

The sensitive nature of healthcare data raises concerns about patient privacy and data security. Ensuring compliance with regulations like HIPAA and GDPR requires robust data protection measures, such as encryption, anonymization, and access controls. Protecting healthcare data from cyberattacks and data breaches is another significant challenge, as healthcare organizations are often targeted by cybercriminals due to the value of the data they hold.

Bias in training data or algorithms can lead to unfair or discriminatory treatment decisions, negatively impacting patient outcomes and trust in IIS. Addressing transparency, interpretability, and fairness in the IIS is essential to ensure ethical decision-making in healthcare.

Healthcare organizations often generate large volumes of data, requiring IIS to be scalable and capable of handling big data efficiently. The ability to adapt to the evolving needs of the healthcare sector, such as new data sources, treatment protocols, and regulations, is critical for the long-term success of IIS.

Resistance from healthcare professionals, administrators, and patients can hinder the adoption of IIS in healthcare settings. Engaging stakeholders and addressing their concerns is crucial for the successful implementation of IIS. Providing education and training on the use and interpretation of IIS outputs can help increase acceptance and trust in the system.

Demonstrating the effectiveness and accuracy of IIS in real-world healthcare settings is a significant challenge. Rigorous evaluation and validation, using metrics like sensitivity, specificity, and positive predictive value, are necessary to establish the system's credibility. Longitudinal studies and clinical trials can help assess the impact of IIS on patient outcomes, cost reduction, and healthcare provider efficiency.

Regulatory frameworks for IIS in healthcare are still evolving, making it challenging for healthcare organizations to navigate the complex landscape of rules and requirements. Ensuring compliance with local and international regulations, such as FDA approval for medical devices and software, is essential to avoid legal and financial repercussions.

While IIS offers promising opportunities for improving the healthcare sector, several challenges need to be addressed to ensure their successful implementation and adoption. Overcoming these challenges will require a collaborative effort from researchers, healthcare providers, policymakers, and other stakeholders.

Now, the future research directions will be discussed in the following part.

6.2 Future Directions

Intelligent Information Systems (IIS) in the healthcare sector have shown great potential for improving patient care, reducing costs, and enhancing operational efficiency. However, there are still many challenges and opportunities for future research in this area. Below, we discuss some possible future research directions for IIS in healthcare:

As machine learning and AI techniques continue to evolve, investigating and incorporating these advanced methods in IIS healthcare applications can lead to more accurate and efficient predictions, decision-making, and resource allocation. Some potential research areas include Deep learning for medical image analysis, Graph neural networks for drug discovery and disease modeling and Transfer learning and domain adaptation for leveraging pre-trained models in healthcare.

The development of interpretable and explainable AI models is crucial for gaining the trust of healthcare professionals and patients, as well as ensuring ethical and transparent decision-making. Future research can focus on: Explainable machine learning models for diagnostics and treatment planning, Techniques to measure and improve the interpretability of AI models and integrating human expertise with AI to create hybrid decision support systems.

IIS can play a key role in advancing personalized and precision medicine by enabling data-driven insights at the individual patient level. Potential research directions include Integrating multi-omics data (genomics, transcriptomics, proteomics, etc.) for better patient characterization, Developing models for patient subtyping and treatment response prediction and AI-based methods for drug repurposing and personalized treatment recommendations.

The development of real-time and adaptive IIS can help healthcare professionals make more informed decisions in dynamic and time-sensitive situations. Future research can explore: Real-time monitoring and alert systems for critical care and remote patient monitoring, Adaptive models that continuously learn and update as new data becomes available and Integrating IIS with Internet of Medical Things (IoMT) devices for real-time data collection and analysis.

Addressing privacy concerns and ensuring data security are critical aspects of IIS in healthcare. Future research can investigate: Federated learning approaches for training AI models on decentralized data, Privacy-preserving techniques, such as differential privacy and secure multiparty computation and Balancing privacy and utility in healthcare AI applications.

To ensure the safe and effective use of IIS in healthcare, rigorous evaluation and validation methods are needed. Future research can focus on: Developing standardized benchmarks and performance metrics for IIS healthcare applications, Investigating the impact of data quality, model uncertainty, and algorithmic bias on IIS performance and Longitudinal studies to assess the real-world impact of IIS on patient outcomes and healthcare efficiency.

For IIS to have a meaningful impact in healthcare, it must be integrated with existing workflows, policies, and regulations. Future research can explore: Identifying and addressing barriers to IIS adoption in healthcare settings, developing strategies for seamless integration of IIS with Electronic Health Records (EHRs) and other healthcare systems and assessing the implications of IIS on healthcare policies, regulations, and guidelines.

By exploring these research directions, the potential of IIS in the healthcare sector can be further harnessed to improve patient outcomes, reduce costs, and drive innovation in medical research and technology.

The following section presents conclusion of this research paper.

7 Conclusion

In conclusion, this research review paper has provided an in-depth analysis of the growing significance of Intelligent Information Systems (IIS) in the healthcare sector. As the industry continues to evolve and face increasing challenges such as rising costs, aging populations, and the need for personalized care, IIS has emerged as a promising solution to address these issues while enhancing patient outcomes and healthcare operations.

The paper has comprehensively discussed various components of IIS, including electronic health records, machine learning algorithms, natural language processing, and computer vision techniques, and their applications in healthcare. Furthermore, the integration of IIS with emerging technologies such as the Internet of Things (IoT) and telemedicine platforms has been examined, showcasing the potential for further innovation and synergies in the field.

A practical framework for implementing IIS in the healthcare sector has been proposed, offering a structured approach to harnessing the power of these advanced technologies and methodologies. This framework not only highlights the different stages involved in the development and deployment of IIS but also emphasizes key considerations such as data privacy, security, ethics, and stakeholder engagement.

Despite the numerous advancements and successes of IIS in healthcare, challenges persist in terms of technical, ethical, and organizational aspects. This paper has identified these challenges and suggested future research directions to address them, paving the way for more effective and efficient implementation of IIS in healthcare settings.

In summary, IIS is poised to revolutionize the healthcare industry by fostering data-driven decision-making, personalized care, and improved operational efficiency. This research review paper has emphasized the transformative potential of IIS in healthcare and underscored the need for ongoing research, collaboration, and innovation to fully realize its benefits and shape a more sustainable and patient-centric future for healthcare.

References

1. Sharda, R., Turban, E., Delen, D., Aronson, J.E., Liang, T.P., King, D.: Business Intelligence and Analytics: Systems for Decision Support. Pearson, London (2014)
2. Raghupathi, W., Raghupathi, V.: Big data analytics in healthcare: promise and potential. Health Inf. Sci. Syst. **2**, 3 (2014)
3. Berner, E., Lande, T.: Overview of Clinical Decision Support Systems, pp. 1–17, July 2016
4. Jiang, F., et al.: Artificial intelligence in healthcare: past, present and future. Stroke Vasc. Neurol. **2**(4), 230–243 (2017)

5. Ali, O., Abdelbaki, W., Shrestha, A., Elbasi, E., Alryalat, M.A.A., Dwivedi, Y.K.: A systematic literature review of artificial intelligence in the healthcare sector: benefits, challenges, methodologies, and functionalities. J. Innov. Knowl.Innov. Knowl. **8**(1), 100333 (2023)
6. Bates, D.W., Saria, S., Ohno-Machado, L., Shah, A., Escobar, G.: Big data in health care: using analytics to identify and manage high-risk and high-cost patients. Health Aff. (Millwood) **33**(7), 1123–1131 (2014)
7. Jha, A.K., et al.: Use of electronic health records in U.S. hospitals. N. Engl. J. Med. **360**(16), 1628–1638 (2009)
8. Vest, J.R., Gamm, L.D.: Health information exchange: persistent challenges and new strategies. J. Am. Med. Inform. Assoc. **17**(3), 288–294 (2010)
9. Kawamoto, K., Houlihan, C.A., Balas, E.A., Lobach, D.F.: Improving clinical practice using clinical decision support systems: a systematic review of trials to identify features critical to success. BMJ **330**(7494), 765 (2005)
10. Holzinger, A., Langs, G., Denk, H., Zatloukal, K., Müller, H.: Causability and explainability of artificial intelligence in medicine. Wiley Interdiscip. Rev. Data Min. Knowl. Discov. **9**(4), e1312 (2019)
11. Jagannatha, A.N., Yu, H.: Bidirectional RNN for medical event detection in electronic health records. Proc. Conf. **2016**, 473–482 (2016)
12. Laranjo, L., et al.: Conversational agents in healthcare: a systematic review. J. Am. Med. Inform. Assoc. **25**(9), 1248–1258 (2018)
13. Kourou, K., Exarchos, T.P., Exarchos, K.P., Karamouzis, M.V., Fotiadis, D.I.: Machine learning applications in cancer prognosis and prediction. Comput. Struct. Biotechnol. J.. Struct. Biotechnol. J. **13**, 8–17 (2015)
14. Davenport, T., Kalakota, R.: The potential for artificial intelligence in healthcare. Future Hosp. J. **6**, 94–98 (2019)
15. Paschou, M., Papadimitiriou, C., Nodarakis, N., Korezelidis, K., Sakkopoulos, E., Tsakalidis, A.: Enhanced healthcare personnel rostering solution using mobile technologies. J. Syst. Softw.Softw. **100**, 44–53 (2015)
16. Khalaf, M., Hussain, A.J., Al-Jumeily, D., Fergus, P., Keenan, R., Radi, N.: A framework to support ubiquitous healthcare monitoring and diagnostic for sickle cell disease. In: Huang, D.-S., Jo, K.-H., Hussain, A. (eds.) ICIC 2015. LNCS, vol. 9226, pp. 665–675. Springer, Cham (2015). https://doi.org/10.1007/978-3-319-22186-1_66
17. Vázquez-Santacruz, E., Portillo-Flores, R., Gamboa-Zúñiga, M.: Towards intelligent hospital devices: Health caring of patients with motor disabilities (2015)
18. Conejar, R.J., Jung, R., Kim, H.-K.: Smart home IP-based U-healthcare monitoring system using mobile technologies. Int. J. Smart Home **10**(10), 283–292 (2016)
19. Alghanim, A.A., Rahman, S.M.M., Hossain, M.A.: Privacy analysis of smart city healthcare services. **2017-January**, 394–398 (2017)
20. Ara, A., Ara, A.: Case study: integrating IoT, streaming analytics and machine learning to improve intelligent diabetes management system, 3179–3182 (2018)
21. Sigwele, T., Hu, Y.F., Ali, M., Hou, J., Susanto, M., Fitriawan, H.: Intelligent and energy efficient mobile smartphone gateway for healthcare smart devices based on 5G (2018)
22. Kaur, J., Mann, K.S.: AI based healthcare platform for real time, predictive and prescriptive analytics. Commun. Comput. Inf. Sci. **805**, 138–149 (2018)
23. Yu, H.Q.: Experimental disease prediction research on combining natural language processing and machine learning, pp. 145–150 (2019)
24. Htet, H., Khaing, S.S., Myint, Y.Y.: tweets sentiment analysis for healthcare on big data processing and iot architecture using maximum entropy classifier. In: Big Data Analysis and Deep Learning Applications, pp. 28–38 (2019)
25. Sahoo, A.K., Mallik, S., Pradhan, C., Mishra, B.S.P., Barik, R.K., Das, H.: Intelligence-based health recommendation system using big data analytics, pp. 227–246 (2019)

26. Mubarakali, A., Bose, S.C., Srinivasan, K., Elsir, A., Elsier, O.: Design a secure and efficient health record transaction utilizing block chain (SEHRTB) algorithm for health record transaction in block chain. J. Ambient Intell. Human. Comput. (2019)
27. Arulanthu, P., Perumal, E.: An intelligent IoT with cloud centric medical decision support system for chronic kidney disease prediction. Int. J. Imaging Syst. Technol. **30**(3), 815–827 (2020)
28. Bolla, S.J., Jyothi, S.: Big data modelling for predicting side-effects of anticancer drugs: a comprehensive approach. Adv. Intell. Syst. Comput.Intell. Syst. Comput. **1037**, 446–456 (2020)
29. Le, D.-N., Parvathy, V.S., Gupta, D., Khanna, A., Rodrigues, J.J.P.C., Shankar, K.: IoT enabled depthwise separable convolution neural network with deep support vector machine for COVID-19 diagnosis and classification. Int. J. Mach. Learn. Cybern.Cybern. **12**(11), 3235–3248 (2021)
30. El Kah, A., Zeroual, I.: A review on applied natural language processing to electronic health records (2021)
31. Idemen, B.T., Sezer, E., Unalir, M.O.: LabHub: a new generation architecture proposal for intelligent healthcare medical laboratories. In: Kahraman, C., CevikOnar, S., Oztaysi, B., Sari, I.U., Cebi, S., Tolga, A.C. (eds.) INFUS 2020. AISC, vol. 1197, pp. 1284–1291. Springer, Cham (2021). https://doi.org/10.1007/978-3-030-51156-2_150
32. Aljabr, A.A., Kumar, K.: Design and implementation of internet of medical things (IoMT) using artificial intelligent for mobile-healthcare. Meas. Sens. **24** (2022)
33. Rehman, M., et al.: Development of an intelligent real-time multiperson respiratory illnesses sensing system using SDR technology. IEEE Sens. J. **22**(19), 18858–18869 (2022)
34. Merabet, A., Ferradji, M.A.: Smart virtual environment to support collaborative medical diagnosis (2022)
35. Aruna, M., Arulkumar, V., Deepa, M., Latha, G.C.P.: Medical healthcare system with hybrid block based predictive models for quality preserving in medical images using machine learning techniques (2022)

Design of a Blockchain-Based Patient Record Tracking System

Huwida E. Said[1](✉), Nedaa B. Al Barghuthi[2], Sulafa M. Badi[3], and Shini Girija[1]

[1] Zayed University, Dubai, United Arab Emirates
{huwida.said,shini.girija}@zu.ac.ae
[2] Higher Colleges of Technology, Sharjah, United Arab Emirates
nalbarghuthi@hct.ac.ae
[3] The British University of Dubai, Dubai, United Arab Emirates
sulafa.badi@buid.ac.ae

Abstract. The major issues in managing patient health records are the security, accessibility, ownership of medical reports, and usability of medical data. To address these challenges, we propose a decentralized, blockchain-based architecture to connect patient health record systems by bringing together several healthcare stakeholders. Patients could grant healthcare professionals temporary access to their data based on a permission-based process. To accomplish this, we proposed employing the Hyperledger blockchain with Non-Fungible Tokens (NFTs) to verify ownership of patient records, track all associated activities, and offer transparency, security, and swift accessibility. We illustrate the system architecture and functionality using comprehensive design diagrams, including flowcharts, Unified Modelling Language (UML) diagrams, and entity diagrams. The design diagrams visually represent the system's structure and procedures, which helps with implementation and possible applications. In this paper, we have primarily emphasized the structural modeling aspects of the proposed system. Overall, this study adds to the expanding body of knowledge about healthcare systems based on blockchain and offers insightful information for academics, professionals, and decision-makers in the sector.

Keywords: Blockchain · Hyperledger · Non-Fungible tokens · patient record tracking

1 Introduction

The healthcare sector is fast advancing technologically and implementing digital patient record management through electronic health records (EHRs) and personal health records (PHRs) to improve accessibility, reduce medical errors, and lower associated costs [1, 2]. These records may contain a wide range of information in detail or summary form, including demographics, medical history, prescription and allergy information, immunization status, test outcomes, radiology pictures, and billing details. A comprehensive view that matches the concept of a patient-records tracking system is produced by this integration of medical information, which integrates demographic, lifestyle, and

A. Souri and S. Bendak (Eds.): IoTHIC 2023, ECPSCI 8, pp. 145–161, 2024.
https://doi.org/10.1007/978-3-031-52787-6_12

behavioral data with EHR. It can significantly improve personalized care and public health decision-making, leading to better health and wellness, but it also presents significant difficulties and risks to security and privacy [3]. The shortcomings of traditional patient record-keeping systems include their susceptibility to cyberattacks [4], the restriction of patients' access to and control over their records [5], the difficulty of obtaining and transferring forms [6], the fragmentation of data among healthcare providers [7], and the absence of real-time updates, which influence comprehensive care and decision-making [8]. By utilizing blockchain technology, healthcare networks can overcome the drawbacks of traditional patient record tracking systems by providing greater confidentiality, patient monitoring, interoperability of data, and real-time access to the latest health records. Blockchain technology has been undergoing advancements and can potentially enhance the existing patient records tracking system based on HER [9, 10]. According to the literature, role-based access control is a standard model used by EHRs [11, 12]. Blockchain technology with permissions could enhance the authorization approach by utilizing smart contracts and attribute-based access control [25]. This enables patient record tracking systems to provide patients with complete ownership of their medical data [26]. Blockchain, which functions as a decentralized database, offers a dependable solution for the issues of poor sharing, ineffectiveness, and weak safety in medical data management [13]. The real-time shared blockchain platform allows data recording, and timestamps are appended to assure immutability [27]. The security of medical data is guaranteed by the blockchain's tamper-resistance [14]. Blockchain members can access data information on the authorized blockchain through access methods [28]. By leveraging the properties mentioned above of blockchain, such as transparency, security, access control, and immutability, it offers a robust and reliable patient record-tracking system [25, 27, 28].

Blockchain platforms such as Ethereum [29], Hyperledger Fabric [30], and Quorum [31] are prominently used for tracking patient records. These platforms provide tamper-proof, secure, decentralized solutions to the problems of keeping private healthcare data. Ethereum-based patient tracking systems have also been considered for their potential advantages in terms of security, openness, and data integrity [15, 16]. But just like any other technology, blockchain-based patient tracking systems have their own set of drawbacks. These include high costs, interoperability problems caused by the lack of an existing standard, scalability issues, privacy concerns, and regulatory compliance [32–34]. These drawbacks have prevented widespread adoption of these systems in the healthcare industry [35]. The significant contribution of this study is to address these challenges associated with blockchain technology by proposing a Hyperledger-fabric-based blockchain patient tracking system with Non-Fungible Token (NFT). Our proposed Hyperledger fabric-based patient tracking solution was chosen over an Ethereum-based system because it is more suited to managing medical records due to its adaptability, scalability, privacy, and anonymity [17]. This study is the first in the area and aims to significantly advance blockchain-based solutions for tracking patient health records globally. This paper presents detailed design diagrams, such as flowcharts, UML diagrams, and entity diagrams, to show the proposed system's architecture and functionality. The design diagrams' visual representation of the system's structure and processes aids in implementation and potential applications. It is important to note that in this paper, we have presented only structural modeling for the proposed system.

The paper's organization is as follows: Sect. 2 provides an in-depth review of the current research pertaining to blockchain-based patient records tracking systems, emphasizing areas where gaps exist and establishing the study's foundational context. In Sect. 3, we delve into the system design of our proposed solution. Section 4 offers a comprehensive discussion of the merits and benefits of our proposed system. Finally, Sect. 5 encapsulates the essence of our research by summarizing the key findings, analyzing their significance, and proposing potential avenues for future research.

2 Blockchain-Based Patient Records Tracking System-Related Works

The blockchain-based patient records tracking system represents a decentralized, peer-to-peer data processing platform that allows for the creation of an open and distributed online database [18, 19]. These databases are made up of blocks of data. Each block contains a timestamp for when it was created, the hash value of the block before it, and references to the patient's medical records and the details of the healthcare provider. The previous block's hash value creates the chain and unchangeable the blockchain [36, 50]. The patient's medical history will be complete, consistent, timely, accurate, and simple to transmit, which will be the main advantage of implementing the blockchain in the patient records tracking system [20].

Additionally, the patient will own their data [37]. Furthermore, as all data insertions are immutable, any modification made to the blockchain is accessible to all patients in the patient network [38]. Because of this, any unauthorized changes are quickly discovered [39]. One of the main advantages of utilizing such an approach is that it does not require a reliable third party and has no single point of failure [21]. Numerous studies [22–25, 48] examined the advantages of using blockchain technology for patient record-tracking systems that authenticate, authorize, view, and access medical records. Nishi et al. [22] described a blockchain-based system that enables the management and security of the patient's data into a single record maintained by the patient, utilizing the Ethereum platform to store the patient's data and carry out operations in a decentralized system using blockchain smart contracts. The patient can use this system to give and revoke any record-specific powers to the authorities quickly. However, costs increase since there are many transactions and data storage. Zabaar et al. [23] proposed blockchain-based architecture, which is built on Hyperledger Fabric, a permissioned distributed ledger solution, and the ledgers and transactions are stored in the cloud. The proposed architecture contributes to these systems' robustness and avoids recorded security limitations in commonly used approaches. The proposed blockchain-based architecture is built on Hyperledger Fabric, a permissioned distributed ledger solution, and the ledgers and transactions are stored in the cloud. The proposed architecture contributes to these systems' robustness and avoids recorded security limitations in commonly used approaches. However, patient control in medical records needs to be specified, which risks the privacy of medical records.

Jamil et al. [24] developed an innovative framework for decentralized healthcare IoT using Hyperledger fabric blockchain-based smart contracts to track patients' vital signs.

Patients can gain from this method in several ways, including global access to medical data at any time and location and a comprehensive, unchangeable history log. However, it has problems with security because the server and the IoT sensors do not authenticate one another, which results in these risks. Kordestani et al. [25] presented HapiChain, an Ethereum blockchain-based system for patient-centric telemedicine. HapiChain uses blockchain technology to enhance medical workflow's security, scalability, and dependability. Although HapiChain is patient-focused, it also aids doctors in saving time and avoiding pointless journeys without compromising the quality of care. Medical records, however, are not accessible everywhere.

It could be observed from the above scholarly work that patients typically need more control over their health data in many current systems. Patients may need help controlling and accessing their records and need more control over how their information is shared with other healthcare professionals or outside parties [40]. Furthermore, data leaks and cyberattacks are more likely to occur in centralized systems [41]. The risk of unauthorized access and data theft grows when vast amounts of patient data are housed in a single database [42]. Finally, existing blockchain-based systems have high costs and energy consumption [43, 47]. Thus, to address these issues, we propose a Hyperledger-based blockchain system with NFTs for global access to patient records. The proposed system transforms how healthcare data is stored and shared internationally. An NFT is a unit of data recorded on a blockchain ledger, and it verifies a digital asset to be unique and, hence, not interchangeable, which may also verify ownership and validity [44]. Blockchain technology offers access control, including NFTs, which improves transparency, eliminates intermediaries' institutional or personal biases, reduces inefficiencies, and ensures accountability. NFTs allow people to regulate who has access to their data and enable the tokenization of all forms of data (such as text, photos, video, and audio) [45]. Giving patients the option to access data only with their consent by doctors or other stakeholders in the patient records tracking system is one potential application for NFTs in this context. NFTs employ smart contracts, self-executing contracts with the terms put directly into the code. This makes it possible to manage data automatically and effectively, lowering the possibility of mistakes and misunderstandings, storing sensitive data securely, and displaying the information that must be shared publicly [46]. In this system, NFTs provide safe, permissioned access to patient records, guaranteeing data privacy and control while facilitating global access [47, 48]. The solution delivers improved data security, tracking of patients, and interoperability by utilizing blockchain technology [49] and NFTs, opening the path for a more effective and internationally connected healthcare ecosystem.

3 System Design

Our main objective is to present the framework of a blockchain-based system for tracking patient records. As a starting point, we developed a demo prototype to showcase and illustrate the proposed patient records tracking system using Hyperledger. This prototype offers a tangible representation of the system's functionality and features.

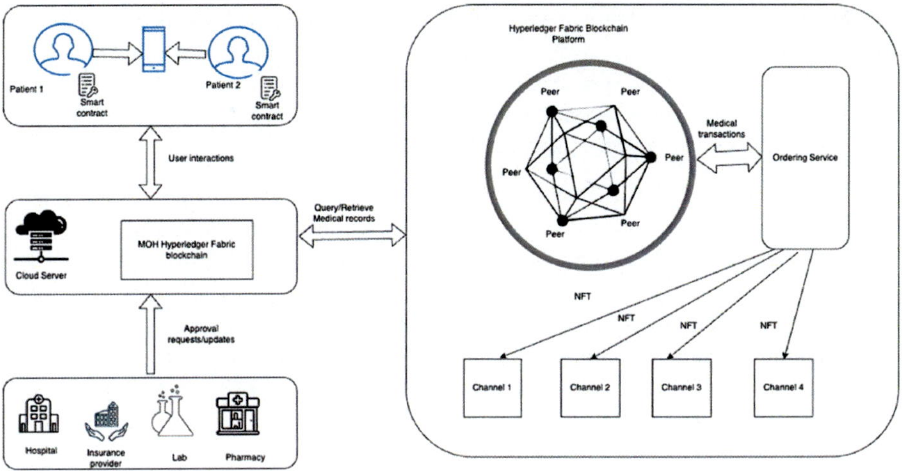

Fig. 1. Hyperledger-based patient records tracking system with NFTs.

3.1 Hyperledger-Based Patient Records Tracking System with NFTs

A secure, decentralized, and permissioned network is built as part of the system design of a blockchain-based medical records tracking system based on Hyperledger Fabric to store and share patient health records among various healthcare industry participants. Figure 1 depicts the design of the Hyperledger-based patient records tracking system with NFTS. Patients, doctors, hospitals, and labs are among the participants who register and receive distinctive NFTs that allow them to communicate with the network according to their assigned tasks. Data privacy and confidentiality are guaranteed by the blockchain's encrypted storage of patient health records. Access controls are governed by smart contracts, ensuring that only parties with permission can access particular patient records. Patients oversee their information and can allow or deny access to their medical records. As a result of the system's support for data interoperability, healthcare providers can exchange data easily.

3.2 Flowchart

The proposed system comprises a centralized healthcare provider portal and a decentralized blockchain-based MoH portal. **Centralized healthcare provider portal**:- At Hospital H, Patient P registers and provides personal and medical data. Through Insurance Provider I, Patient P requests their medical records. The request is checked against predetermined criteria by Insurance Provider I. The proposal is turned down if the conditions are not satisfied. If not, it moves on to the following phase. When the request is approved, Hospital H accepts it using the patient's Emirates ID as a distinctive identification. The patient's blockchain-based health record can be connected to the Emirates ID to ensure accurate identification. At Hospital H, Patient P receives the required consultation. Additional lab requests are handled appropriately if necessary. Examining the lab and consultation requests made by Hospital H is Insurance Provider I. The transactions are carried out under the insurance coverage if the provider approves the bids. However, the patient will be liable for the cost if their demands are rejected. Hospital H communicates with the Ministry of Health (MoH) and records all committed transactions on the blockchain, such as consultation reports, prescriptions, and lab results. The flowchart of the centralized healthcare provider portal is shown in Fig. 2.

Decentralized Blockchain-Based MoH Portal:- The flowchart of working a decentralized blockchain network for tracking patient records l is shown in Fig. 3. The steps in a decentralized blockchain network for tracking patient records are as follows:

- *Registration: On the blockchain network, the MoH network administrator registers healthcare organizations (hospitals, clinics, labs, and pharmacies).*
- *Data Storage: Hospital H interacts with the Ministry of Health (MoH) and safely records every committed transaction, including prescriptions, test results, and reports from consultations, on the blockchain.*
- *Verification: To ensure data accuracy and authenticity, the MoH checks the information recorded in the blockchain using the patient's Emirates ID as the key.*
- *Issuance of a Non-Fungible Certificate (NFC): Following completing the verification, the patient is given a Non-Fungible Certificate (NFC) by the MoH. This NFC is a digital token for the patient's verified and authorized medical records.*
- *International Usability: Hospitals in other nations can accept the NFC certificate. The NFC is authenticated when it is presented to guarantee its reliability.*
- *Authorized Access: With the patient's permission and using the blockchain, authorized healthcare providers can safely access the patient's records. On the blockchain, smart contracts are created and stored, outlining criteria like the requirement of patient approval to access the documents.*
- *Hospital-Specific Record Tracking: To ensure data security and privacy, each Hospital can only track and access the records of its patients.*
- *Doctor Access: During the patient visit and within a predetermined follow-up period, such as seven days, doctors have access to the patient's records, ensuring quick access to pertinent information for appropriate care.*
- *Insurance Company Access: To ensure control over data sharing, other insurance companies can only access a patient's medical records from the blockchain with the patient's explicit consent.*

3.3 Use Case Diagram

As part of the requirements analysis and design process for the ongoing research, we have developed a Unified Modelling Language (UML) use case diagram. This diagram captures the steps that lead to object identification and the formation of complete tasks or transactions within the proposed application. The use case starts as a means of capturing the primary functional objectives and the driving force behind creating the architectural framework for a system that facilitates requirement coverage [31]. The main actors identified in the centralized healthcare provider portal are the Hospital, patient, and insurance provider. The use case diagram of the centralized healthcare provider portal is shown in Fig. 4. The prominent use cases identified for the portal are explained below:

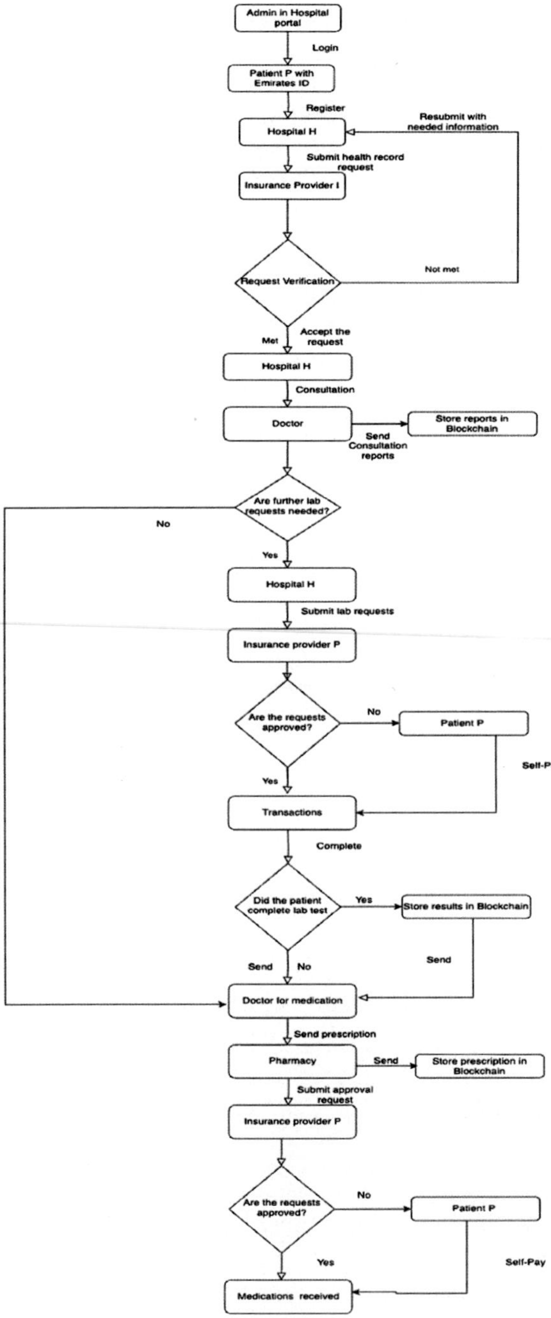

Fig. 2. Flowchart of centralized healthcare provider portal

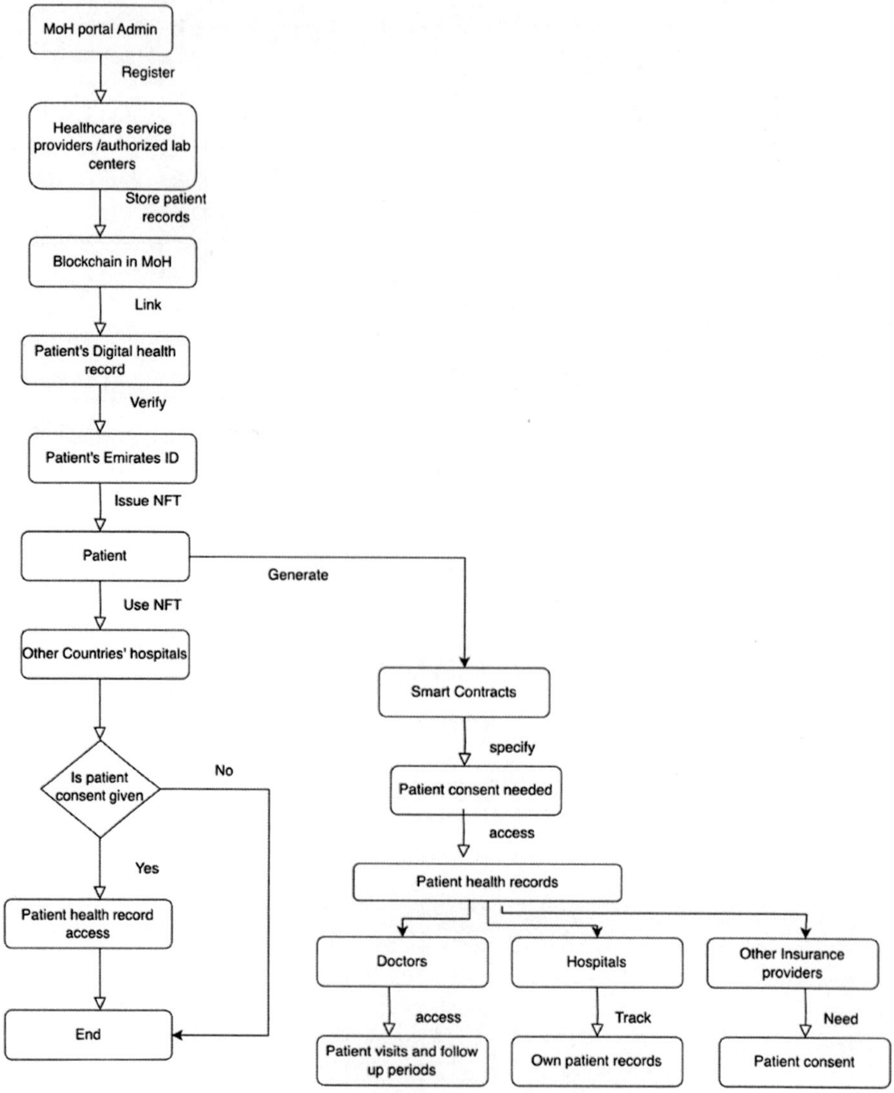

Fig. 3. Flowchart for the decentralized blockchain-based MoH's portal.

- *Register at Hospital: Patient P registers at Hospital H.*
- *Submit Health Record Request:- Hospital H submits an approval request to Insurance Provider I.*
- *Verify Health Record Request: Insurance Provider I review the request regarding predetermined standards.*
- *Accept Health Record Request: When a patient's health record request is approved, Hospital H accepts it and connects it to the patient's blockchain-based health record.*
- *Consultation:- Patient P receives the required consultation at Hospital H.*
- *Process Lab Requests: Hospital H processes lab requests if necessary.*

- *Review Lab Requests: Insurance Provider I review the consultation and lab requests made by Hospital H.*
- *Approve Requests: Insurance Provider: If they meet the insurance coverage, I approve the requests.*
- *Store Transactions on Blockchain: Hospital H stores all committed transactions, including consultation reports, prescriptions, and lab results, in the blockchain of the decentralized MoH portal.*

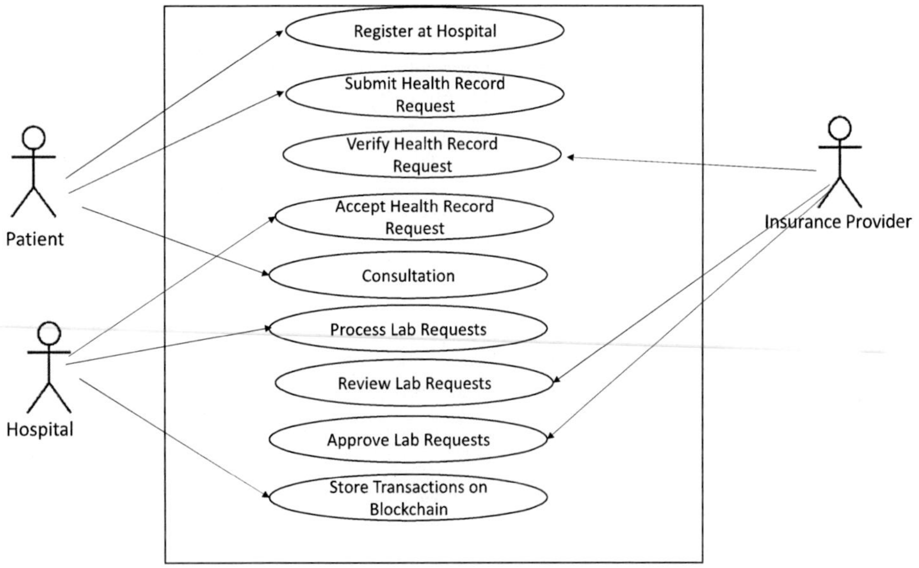

Fig. 4. Use case diagram of centralized healthcare provider portal.

The main actors identified in the decentralized blockchain-based MoH portal are the patient, Hospital, insurance Provider, admin, doctor, and MoH. The use case diagram of the decentralized blockchain-based MoH portal is shown in Fig. 5. The primary use case identified is given below:

- *Registration of healthcare entities: Admin registers healthcare entities (hospitals, clinics, labs, pharmacies) on the blockchain network.*
- *Verify records: Verification by MoH: MoH verifies the details stored in the blockchain using the patient's Emirates ID as the key.*
- *Issue Digital Attested Certificate (NFC): MoH issues the patient a digital attested certificate (NFC) once verification is complete. The NFC is a digital token representing the patient's authorized and validated health records.*
- *Generate smart contracts: Smart contracts are generated and stored on the blockchain.*
- *Use NFC in other countries for authentication: The NFC certificate can be used in hospitals in other countries to access patient records.*

- *Give consent to access records: Conditions, such as patient consent, are stored in the smart contracts to control access to records.*
- *Track and access patient records: Every Hospital can track and access only its patients' records.*
- *Access records during patient visits and follow-up periods:- Doctors can access patient records during the patient's visit and within a specified follow-up period (e.g., seven days).*
- *Access records with patient consent:- Other insurance companies can access medical records from the blockchain, but only with the patient's consent.*

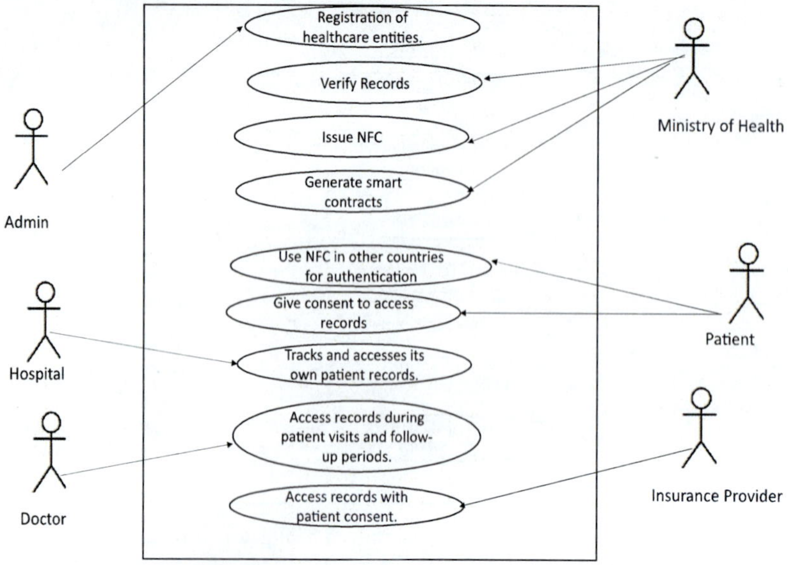

Fig. 5. Use-case diagram of decentralized blockchain-based MoH portal.

3.4 Sequence Diagram

The sequence diagram is generally used to depict object interactions in the order in which they occur [32]. Sequence diagrams are frequently developed from use cases. Sequence diagrams can document the current interactions between items in an existing system and their usage in designing new systems. The use case diagram of the decentralized blockchain-based MoH portal is shown in Fig. 6.

- *The sequence begins with Patient P registering at Hospital H by submitting their personal and medical information.*
- *Hospital H then submits a request for their health records through Insurance Provider I.*
- *Insurance Provider: I verify the request against predefined criteria. If the requirements are unmet, the request is rejected, and Patient P needs to resubmit the bid.*

- *Once approved, Hospital H accepts the request using the patient's Emirates ID as a unique identifier. The Emirates ID is linked to the patient's blockchain-based health record, ensuring proper identification.*
- *Patient P undergoes the necessary consultation at Hospital H. If further lab requests are required, they are processed accordingly.*
- *Insurance Provider: I reviewed the consultation and lab requests made by Hospital H. The transactions are completed if the proposals are approved based on the insurance coverage. However, if the requests are not approved, the patient will be responsible for the payment.*
- *Hospital H communicates with the Ministry of Health (MoH) and stores all committed transactions on the blockchain, including consultation reports, prescriptions, and lab results. These transactions are linked to the patient's digital health record.*

The use case diagram of the decentralized blockchain-based MoH portal is shown in Fig. 7. The primary sequence of events in the decentralized blockchain-based MoH portal are listed below:-

- *The sequence starts with the admin registering healthcare entities on the blockchain network, such as hospitals, clinics, labs, and pharmacies.*
- *Hospital H communicates with the Ministry of Health (MoH) to establish a connection and exchange information.*
- *Hospital H stores committed transactions, including consultation reports, prescriptions, and lab results, on the blockchain.*
- *Hospital H links these transactions to the patient's digital health record, ensuring the data is associated with the correct patient.*
- *The Ministry of Health (MoH) verifies the details in the blockchain using the patient's Emirates ID as the key. This verification ensures the integrity and authenticity of the patient's records.*
- *Once the verification is complete, the MoH issues the patient a digitally attested certificate (NFC). This certificate is a digital token representing the patient's authorized and validated health records.*
- *The patient can use the NFC certificate in hospitals located in other countries, allowing for international usage.*
- *When the NFC certificate is presented, it is authenticated, ensuring its validity and integrity.*
- *Authorized healthcare providers, such as doctors, can securely access the patient's records through the blockchain based on the patient's consent. This access occurs during the patient's visit and within a specified follow-up period (e.g., seven days).*
- *The smart contracts stored on the blockchain include access conditions, such as patient consent, which control the access to the records.*
- *Each Hospital can track and access only its patients' records, ensuring data privacy and segregation between healthcare providers.*
- *Other insurance companies can access medical records from the blockchain only with the patient's consent. This ensures that the patient retains control over their data and can manage access rights.*

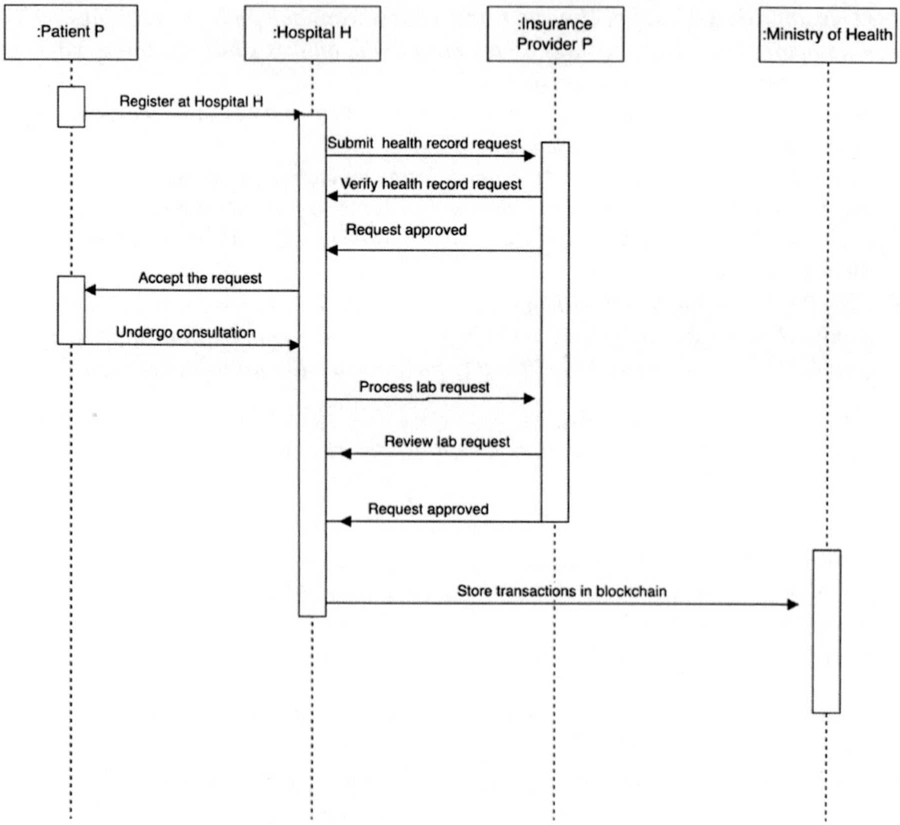

Fig. 6. Sequence diagram of centralized healthcare provider portal.

4 Discussion

The proposed Hyperledger-based patient records tracking systems provide higher trust, decentralization, transparency, privacy, security, data integrity, deployment, modularity, and scalability than other blockchain platforms such as Ethereum and Quorum. These designs may be essential building blocks for developing private permissioned blockchain ecosystems where stakeholders in patient tracking systems are registered with, under the control of, and subject to regulatory oversight by a governing body—MoH. Some of the notable advantages include:

- **High Usability:** *An advantage of the proposed Hyperledger-based Patient Record System is its user-friendly design, which simplifies interactions for administrators, patients, and healthcare professionals, fostering seamless communication. This system prioritizes usability by incorporating accessibility features and providing comprehensive user training. Moreover, it benefits from continuous improvement as user feedback is actively collected and iterative enhancements are made based on their* *valuable suggestions. This user-centric approach ensures that the system remains highly usable and efficient, enhancing the overall healthcare experience.*

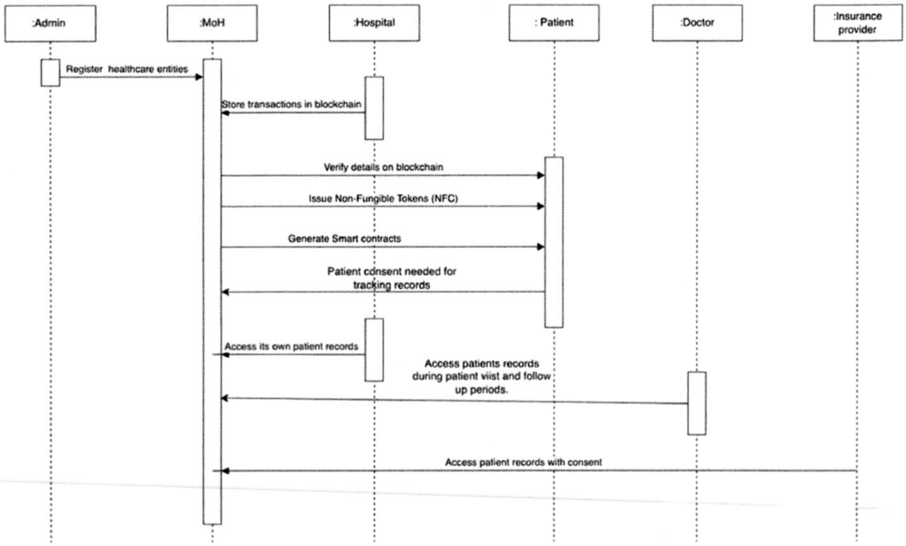

Fig. 7. Sequence diagram of decentralized blockchain-based MoH portal.

- **Data security and privacy:** *The Hyperledger Fabric architecture suggested in this paper offers a preliminary design for a patient record tracking system. It allows for identifying various system stakeholders and establishing their relationships via multiple channels to maximize data security, privacy, and confidentiality. Data security is ensured by blockchain technology's decentralization and cryptographic hashing.*
- **Optimized efficiency:** *The proposed system's focus on operational efficiency is one of its benefits. The responsiveness of healthcare services is improved by quick transaction processing, which guarantees prompt updates to patient records and access rights. The system's storage and processing resource optimization lowers operating costs while also adhering to environmentally sustainable standards.*
- **Interoperability:** *The current blockchain-based solutions are not fully interoperable because there are no standardized methods to facilitate integration, flexibility, and implementation. The proposed system addresses the need for interoperability while guaranteeing optimal scalability and adaptability to enable internal and external communication among healthcare practitioners and access to relevant patient data from various locations and systems.*
- **Patient Control and Consent:** *The blockchain network's smart contracts allow patients to manage who has access to their records. Patients can explicitly consent to doctors and insurance providers to access data, protecting their privacy and the ownership of their data.*

- **International Usability:** *Patients may access their authorized medical records at hospitals abroad using the NFC token granted by the MoH. This makes care more seamless and gives healthcare professionals worldwide access to vital patient data when needed.*
- **Trust**: *MoH uses the patient's Emirates ID as the key to validate patient records. The accuracy and legitimacy of the data recorded on the blockchain are ensured through this verification procedure, boosting trust in the healthcare system.*
- **Improved Patient Care:** *With safe and convenient access to patient records, healthcare professionals may make quicker, more informed decisions that result in better patient outcomes.*
- **Data accuracy and consistency:** *Data accuracy and consistency are improved by the decentralized and synchronized updating of data on the blockchain, which reduces the likelihood of replication of data, inconsistencies, or faults.*
- **Cost of implementation:** *Most existing systems confront one of the most significant difficulties in implementation and energy costs. When it comes to transaction execution, the current platforms and legacy software systems are inefficient and centralized, which results in high implementation and maintenance costs. Because of its various consensus methods, Hyperledger Fabric can complete more than 3500 transactions per second while using substantially less power than Ethereum.*

5 Conclusion

In conclusion, this research proposes a decentralized, blockchain-based architecture for patient health record systems, offering an innovative approach to address essential concerns in the healthcare technology field. This approach uses Non-Fungible Tokens (NFTs) and Hyperledger blockchain to ensure safe, open, and accessible patient data management. The suggested architecture unites all parties involved in the healthcare system. It allows patients to temporarily authorize access to their data through a permission-based system, improving data ownership and control. To guarantee data integrity and accountability, NFTs are used to verify ownership and track all activity related to patient records. The thorough design diagrams offered in this paper make comprehending the system's functioning and structure easier, making implementation and prospective applications easier. The main limitations of the proposed system are inefficiency and cost associated with replacing existing systems for implementing NFTs, coupled with the need for more technical experts proficient in NFT technology in the healthcare industry. Additionally, the demanding storage requirements of NFTs, particularly when dealing with significant patient health information, may exceed the capacity of the current infrastructure and cause issues with data management and accessibility.

This study adds important knowledge to the increasing body of research on blockchain-based healthcare systems and provides academics, healthcare workers, and industry decision-makers with helpful advice. Adopting this innovative design might put healthcare organizations ahead of the competition and promote better patient care and data management in the constantly evolving healthcare IT ecosystem. Establishing comprehensive policies and industry standards will be essential for the widespread adoption of blockchain and NFTs in healthcare, necessitating further research to ensure alignment with governmental rules and regulations, ultimately fostering a secure and compliant healthcare data ecosystem.

References

1. Cernian, A., Tiganoaia, B., Sacala, I., Pavel, A., Iftemi, A.: Patientdatachain: a blockchain-based approach to integrate personal health records. Sensors **20**(22), 6538 (2020)
2. Roehrs, A., Da Costa, C.A., da Rosa Righi, R., De Oliveira, K.S.F.: Personal health records: a systematic literature review. J. Med. Internet Res. **19**(1), e5876 (2017)
3. Heart, T., Ben-Assuli, O., Shabtai, I.: A review of PHR, EMR and EHR integration: a more personalized healthcare and public health policy. Health Policy Technol. **6**(1), 20–25 (2017)
4. Adlam, R., Haskins, B.: A permissioned blockchain approach to the authorization process in electronic health records. In: 2019 International Multidisciplinary Information Technology and Engineering Conference (IMITEC), pp. 1–8. IEEE, November 2019
5. van Mens, H.J., Duijm, R.D., Nienhuis, R., de Keizer, N.F., Cornet, R.: Determinants and outcomes of patient access to medical records: systematic review of systematic reviews. Int. J. Med. Inform. **129**, 226–233 (2019)
6. Luster, J., Yanagawa, F.S., Bendas, C., Ramirez, C.L., Cipolla, J., Stawicki, S.P.: Interhospital transfers: managing competing priorities while ensuring patient safety. In: Vignettes in Patient Safety, vol. 2. IntechOpen (2017)
7. Noest, S., et al.: Involving patients in detecting quality gaps in a fragmented healthcare system: development of a questionnaire for Patients' Experiences Across Health Care Sectors (PEACS). Int. J. Qual. Health Care **26**(3), 240–249 (2014)
8. Schwab, P., et al.: Real-time prediction of COVID-19-related mortality using electronic health records. Nat. Commun. **12**(1), 1058 (2021)
9. Sun, Z., Han, D., Li, D., Wang, X., Chang, C.C., Wu, Z.: A blockchain-based secure storage scheme for medical information. EURASIP J. Wirel. Commun. Netw. **2022**(1), 40 (2022)
10. Kumar, K.A.: Blockchain framework for medical healthcare records. Turk. J. Comput. Math. Educ. (TURCOMAT) **12**(9), 7–12 (2021)
11. Zhang, R., Liu, L., Xue, R.: Role-based and time-bound access and management of EHR data. Secur. Commun. Netw. **7**(6), 994–1015 (2014)
12. de Carvalho Junior, M.A., Bandiera-Paiva, P.: Health information system role-based access control current security trends and challenges. J. Healthc. Eng. (2018)
13. Pradhan, N.R., Rout, S.S., Singh, A.P.: Blockchain-based smart healthcare system for chronic–illness patient monitoring. In: 2020 3rd International Conference on Energy, Power and Environment: Towards Clean Energy Technologies, pp. 1–6. IEEE, March 2021
14. Goel, U., Ruhl, R., Zavarsky, P.: Using healthcare authority and patient blockchains to develop a tamper-proof record tracking system. In: 2019 IEEE 5th International Conference on Big Data Security on Cloud (BigDataSecurity), IEEE International Conference on High Performance and Smart Computing,(HPSC) and IEEE International Conference on Intelligent Data and Security (IDS), pp. 25–30. IEEE, May 2019
15. Jabarulla, M.Y., Lee, H.N.: Blockchain-based distributed patient-centric image management system. Appl. Sci. **11**(1), 196 (2020)
16. Hasan, A., Abrar, M., Nitu, S.H., Saraswathi, A.: An innovative healthcare records management system with ethereum and IPFS (2023)
17. Díaz, Á., Kaschel, H.: Scalable electronic health record management system using a dual-channel blockchain hyperledger fabric. Systems **11**(7), 346 (2023)
18. Esposito, C., De Santis, A., Tortora, G., Chang, H., Choo, K.K.R.: Blockchain: a panacea for healthcare cloud-based data security and privacy? IEEE Cloud Comput. **5**(1), 31–37 (2018)
19. Kaur, H., Alam, M.A., Jameel, R., Mourya, A.K., Chang, V.: A proposed solution and future direction for blockchain-based heterogeneous medicare data in cloud environment. J. Med. Syst. **42**, 1–11 (2018)

20. Hölbl, M., Kompara, M., Kamišalić, A., Nemec Zlatolas, L.: A systematic review of the use of blockchain in healthcare. Symmetry **10**(10), 470 (2018)
21. Al-Ahmadi, B., Sharaf, S.: Blockchain-based remote patient monitoring system. J. King Abdulaziz Univ. Comput. Inf. Technol. Sci. **8**(2), 111–118 (2019)
22. Nishi, F.K., et al.: Electronic healthcare data record security using blockchain and smart contracts. J. Sens. **2022**, 1–22 (2022)
23. Zaabar, B., Cheikhrouhou, O., Ammi, M., Awad, A.I., Abid, M.: Secure and privacy-aware blockchain-based remote patient monitoring system for the Internet of Healthcare things. In: 2021 17th International Conference on Wireless and Mobile Computing, Networking and Communications (WiMob), pp. 200–205. IEEE, October 2021
24. Jamil, F., Ahmad, S., Iqbal, N., Kim, D.H.: Towards remote monitoring of patient vital signs based on IoT-based blockchain integrity management platforms in smart hospitals. Sensors **20**(8), 2195 (2020)
25. Zhonghua, C., Goyal, S.B., Rajawat, A.S.: Smart contracts attribute-based access control model for security & privacy of IoT system using blockchain and edge computing. J. Supercomput. 1–30 (2023)
26. Deepa, V.V., Thamotharan, B., Mahto, D., Rajendiran, P., Sriram, A.L., Chandramohan, K.: Smart embedded health monitoring system and secure electronic health record (EHR) transactions using blockchain technology. Soft Comput. 1–16 (2023)
27. Alam, S., et al.: An overview of blockchain and IoT integration for monitoring secure and reliable health records. Sustainability **15**(7), 5660 (2023)
28. Xu, S., Zhang, C., Wang, L., Zhang, S., Shao, W.: A cross data center access control model by constructing GAS on blockchain. In: 2022 IEEE 28th International Conference on Parallel and Distributed Systems (ICPADS), pp. 312–321. IEEE, January 2023
29. Ucbas, Y., Eleyan, A., Hammoudeh, M., Alohaly, M.: Performance and scalability analysis of ethereum and hyperledger fabric. IEEE Access (2023)
30. Sarkar, S.: Blockchain for combating pharmaceutical drug counterfeiting and cold chain distribution. Asian J. Res. Com. Sci **16**(3), 156–166 (2023)
31. Hegde, P., Maddikunta, P.K.R.: Amalgamation of blockchain with resource-constrained IoT devices for Healthcare applications–state of art, challenges and future directions. Int. J. Cogn. Comput. Eng. (2023)
32. Xosrov, C.C.: Use cases for blockchain in the development of digital health. Endless Light Sci. (июнь), 590–593 (2023)
33. Ray, S., Korchagina, E.V., Nikam, R.U., Singhal, R.K.: A Blockchain-based secure healthcare solution for poverty-led economy of IoMT under industry 5.0. In: Inclusive Developments Through Socio-economic Indicators: New Theoretical and Empirical Insights, pp. 269–280. Emerald Publishing Limited (2023)
34. Pathak, R., Soni, B., Muppalaneni, N.B.: Role of blockchain in health care: a comprehensive study. In: Gunjan, V.K., Zurada, J.M. (eds.) Proceedings of 3rd International Conference on Recent Trends in Machine Learning, IoT, Smart Cities and Applications. LNNS, vol. 540, pp. 137–154. Springer, Singapore (2023). https://doi.org/10.1007/978-981-19-6088-8_13
35. Jeenath Laila, N., Devasurithi, S.: Transforming healthcare: exploring blockchain-based patient record management systems for secure and efficient data sharing
36. Panda, K., Mazumder, A.: Blockchain-powered supply chain management for kidney organ preservation. arXiv preprint arXiv:2308.11169 (2023)
37. Meisami, S., Meisami, S., Yousefi, M., Aref, M.R.: Combining blockchain and IOT for decentralized healthcare data management. arXiv preprint arXiv:2304.00127 (2023)
38. Patel, H., Soans, M., Moorthy, P., Murudkar, M., Das, S.: Swasthya-an EHR built on blockchain. In: 2023 3rd International Conference on Intelligent Technologies (CONIT), pp. 1–7. IEEE, June 2023

39. Cerchione, R., Centobelli, P., Riccio, E., Abbate, S., Oropallo, E.: Blockchain's coming to hospitals to digitalize healthcare services: designing a distributed electronic health record ecosystem: technovation, **120**, 102480 (2023)
40. Ranjan, M.K., Sattar, A.M., Tiwari, S.K.: Blockchain in healthcare systems: an industry prospective study. In: Contemporary Applications of Data Fusion for Advanced Healthcare Informatics, pp. 238–259. IGI Global (2023)
41. Kumar, K.P., Varma, N.H., Devisree, N., Ali, M.S.: Implementation of associative service recommendation scheme applying Sha256 algorithm through blockchain. J. Surv. Fisher. Sci. **10**(2S), 2741–2747 (2023)
42. Javaid, M., Haleem, A., Singh, R.P., Suman, R.: Towards insighting cybersecurity for healthcare domains: a comprehensive review of recent practices and trends. Cyber Secur. Appl. 100016 (2023)
43. Karumba, S., Sethuvenkatraman, S., Dedeoglu, V., Jurdak, R., Kanhere, S.S.: Barriers to blockchain-based decentralized energy trading: a systematic review. Int. J. Sustain. Energ. **42**(1), 41–71 (2023)
44. Yaghy, A., et al.: The potential use of non-fungible tokens (NFTs) in healthcare and medical research. PLOS Digit. Health **2**(7), e0000312 (2023)
45. Teo, Z.L., Ting, D.S.W.: Non-fungible tokens for the management of health data. Nat. Med. **29**(2), 287–288 (2023)
46. Hammi, B., Zeadally, S., Perez, A.J.: Non-fungible tokens: a review. IEEE Internet Things Mag. **6**(1), 46–50 (2023)
47. Said, H., Al Barghuthi, N., Badi, S., Girija, S.: How can blockchain technology be used to manage the COVID-19 vaccine supply chain? A systematic literature review and future research directions. In: Yang, XS., Sherratt, R.S., Dey, N., Joshi, A. (eds.) ICICT 2023. LNNS, vol. 695, pp. 399–418. Springer, Singapore (2024). https://doi.org/10.1007/978-981-99-3043-2_31
48. Al Barghuthi, N., Said, H.E., Badi, S.M., Girija, S.: Security risk assessment of blockchain-based patient health record systems. In: Papadaki, M., Rupino da Cunha, P., Themistocleous, M., Christodoulou, K. (eds.) EMCIS 2022. LNBIP, vol. 464, pp. 477–496. Springer, Cham (2023). https://doi.org/10.1007/978-3-031-30694-5_35
49. Al Barghuthi, N., Ncube, C., Said, H.: State of art of the effectiveness in adopting blockchain technology - UAE survey study. In: Sixth HCT Information Technology Trends (ITT), Ras Al Khaimah, United Arab Emirates, pp. 54–59 (2019). https://doi.org/10.1109/ITT48889.2019.9075108
50. AlTaei, M., Al Barghuthi, N., Mahmoud, Q.H., Barghuthi, S.A., Said, H.: Blockchain for UAE organizations: insights from CIOs with opportunities and challenges. In: 2018 International Conference on Innovations in Information Technology (IIT), Al Ain, United Arab Emirates, pp. 157–162 (2018). https://doi.org/10.1109/INNOVATIONS.2018.8606033

IoT Networks and Online Image Processing in IMU-Based Gait Analysis

Bora Ayvaz[1](✉), Hakan İlikçi[2], Fuat Bilgili[2], and Ali Fuat Ergenç[1]

[1] Department of Control and Automation Engineering, Faculty of Electrical and Electronics Engineering, Istanbul Technical University, Istanbul, Turkey
{ayvazb17,ergenca}@itu.edu.tr

[2] Department of Orthopedic and Biomedical Neurotechnology, Istanbul Faculty of Medicine, Istanbul University, Istanbul, Turkey
hakan.ilikci@ogr.iu.edu.tr, fuat.bilgili@istanbul.edu.tr

Abstract. Gait analysis is a comprehensive anatomical methodology, involves neural, musculoskeletal, and cardiorespiratory systems, utilized for diverse clinical objectives. The analysis techniques in gait analysis has evolved due to biomedical and electrical-electronic engineering progress, transitioning away from conventional visual techniques toward integrated solutions merging sensor and image processing methods. Integration of the Internet of Things technologies into this field has allowed the use of sensor and image processing techniques together in gait analysis which helped clinicals to follow the process more efficiently and to obtaining the results faster. This study presents an IoT-infrastructured system for gait analysis and explains the used IoT technologies, sensor fusion methods, sensor-camera calibration techniques, and an interface for clinical data monitoring. In addition, the actual application and experiment results for a patient are compared with the medical gold standard results of the same patient and the results produced by the sensor-camera integration at various rates are shown in this paper. Experiment results show that the developed gait analysis system provides correlated outputs with same patient's golden standart results without the effect of camera synchronization. The camera synchronization improves the gait data in various joints for a interval of integration while it does not for other cases.

Keywords: Internet of Things · Gait Analysis · Image Processing · Sensor Fusion · MQTT · IMU · Network

1 Introduction

Gait analysis is a technique utilized in various clinical applications to diagnose and monitor specific diseases, assess athletic performance, prevent injuries, monitor the rehabilitation process, and evaluate the effectiveness of treatments. Gait analysis enables users to determine the phases of walking, detect the kinematic and kinetic parameters of human walking events, and assess musculo-skeletal functions. Gait analysis has found applications in sports, rehabilitation, and healthcare diagnostics as a result [1].

A. Souri and S. Bendak (Eds.): IoTHIC 2023, ECPSCI 8, pp. 162–177, 2024.
https://doi.org/10.1007/978-3-031-52787-6_13

Gait analysis used to carried out by medical professionals through the utilization of visual observations. However, recent advancements in biomedical engineering have introduced wearable sensor systems equipped with inertial measurement units (IMUs) as a more suitable, user-friendly and reliable method for gait analysis. Wearable sensors commonly placed on joints enable extended periods of gait monitoring [2].

Image processing technologies are frequently used obtaining gait analysis data alongside sensors. These image processing methods are executed by placing various points of active or passive markers [3]. The systems considered as the medical gold standard solely rely on image data even though measurement techniques that combine sensor and image technologies have been developed [4]. Image processing-based gait analysis systems are typically conducted offline using recorded video footage of the individual walking with markers. This results in delays in obtaining analysis results over extended periods. The aim of this study is to develop a gait analysis system that integrates Internet of Things (IoT) networks into an IMU-based gait analysis system. This integration would allow for the utilization of both real-time sensor data and online image processing data, enabling the development of a gait analysis system capable of providing instantaneous visualization and short-term analysis results.

This paper is organized into seven sections. The second section, following the introduction, explains gait analysis and its methodology, while the third section details the infrastructure used in the system. The fourth explains the methods used in data Synchronization and pose estimation. The fifth section covers the application of the developed system, the sixth examines the effects of camera calibrations and finally, the seventh section presents the conclusions.

1.1 Literature Review

Research on the development of gait analysis systems primarily focuses on advancing sensor and image processing technologies. Stefanović developed a measurement unit consist of four accelerometers and four load cells to gather data during walking and fed collected data into an intelligent fuzzy inference system governed by predefined fuzzy rules in the scope of his study at 2009 [9].

A calibration method was introduced to compensates positional and magnetic errors in accelerometer and magnetometer data within gait analysis systems in a study conducted by Qui and Lui in 2018. Additionally, they presented a PI controller-based filter design for the fusion of these sensors [10].

Bersamira et al. developed an alternative system to the Vicon Motion Capture (Vicon MoCap) system, which considered as medical golden standart for gait analysis but is costly and difficult to access in a study conducted in 2019. The system was developed by collecting data from depth-sensing cameras and IMU sensors and then synthesizing the data with a deep learning algorithm called Bayesian Regularization Artificial Neural Network (BRANN). The synthesized data achieved a similar level of accuracy when compared to the data obtained from the Vicon MoCap system. This study showed that deep learning algorithms could replace the Vicon MoCap system [4].

The studies of developing gait analysis systems for daily life in personal environments are continuing while majority of applications have developed for clinical usage and clinical environments. The most common limitations for daily life gait analysis systems are the lack of standardization in data capturing methods, database conditions and fusion algorithms [5]. There are several approaches for daily life gait analysis using wearable shoe-based hardware, floor-based walking paths and motion capturing with smartphone camera. Zhang et al. explains the usage of flexible wearable triboelectric sensors in gait detection systems [6]. Moreover Young, Mason, Morris, Stuart and Godfrey suggest markerless motion capture gait analysis using single smartphone camera integrated with internet of things for daily life analysis in their study at 2023 [7]. They also explain the methods of IoT based gait analysis in daily life environments in their study at 2023 [5]. Hahm and Anthony suggest a in home gait analysis systems that uses a combination of wearable sensors and floor-based gait path that provides better gait phase detection [8].

2 Gait Analysis System Design

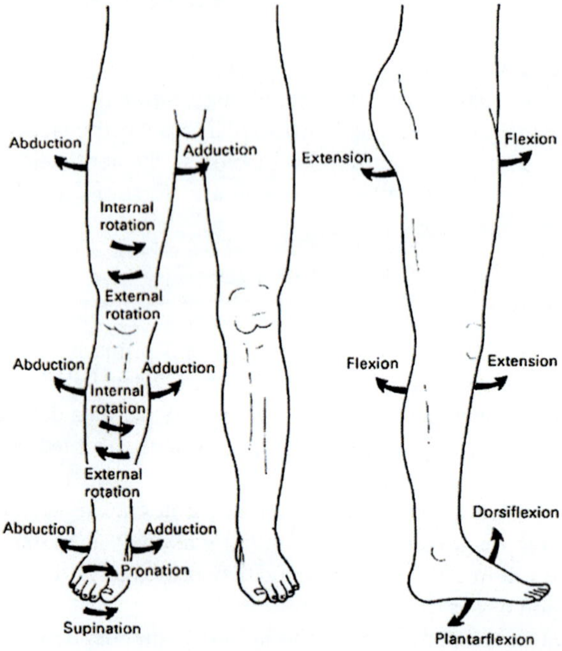

Fig. 1. Sub-body major joint movements [11].

Whittle defined the six main sub-body joint movements, as shown in Fig. 1 [11]. All of these movements must be able to be detected online in the gait analysis system using both IMU sensors and live camera images. The systems established to provide that can be examined under the titles of sensor infrastructure, image processing method and IoT and server infrastructure.

2.1 Sensor Infrastructure

Three IMU sensors were placed at each joint point in a single leg, for a total of six sensors in order to fully detect the joint movements shown in Fig. 1. Both linear acceleration and angular velocity measurements has been carried out using these sensors. Figure 2 shows the IMU sensors placed on the leg and the microcontroller. The microcontroller was chosen to have a wireless network connection. This feature allows microcontroller to provide sensor data communication over a wireless network.

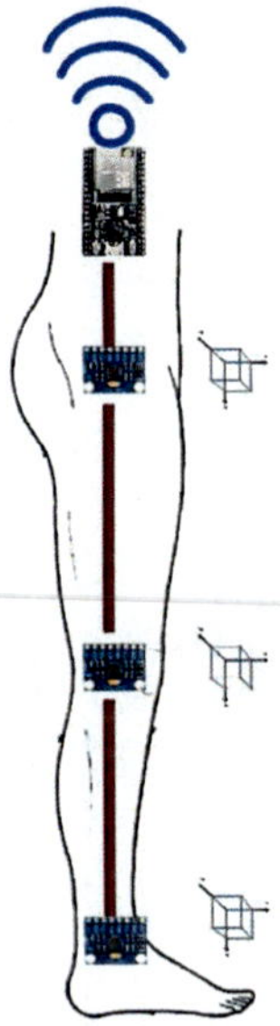

Fig. 2. Positioning of IMU sensors and the microcontroller.

2.2 Image Processing Method

The purpose of using image processing in the system is to support the measurements of IMU sensors with visually calculated 3D acceleration measurements at each joint. An image processing method that can track markers has been developed for this purpose which can be examined under the titles of marker selection and image processing algorithm.

Marker Selection. A suitable marker should be selected for this system which measures linear accelerations of each marker placed on the leg with marker tracking algorithms. The main features that the marker should have include are having a special identity (ID), having fixed and known real-world dimensions, and being easy to detect.

The "AruCo Marker" has chosen as the most suitable marker for camera- assisted - IMU-based gait analysis application considering these features. Methods for creating and detecting AruCo markers are described in a 2014 study by Garrido-Jurado and

Muñoz-Salinas [12]. Each of the AruCo markers has a different ID and the edge lengths of each marker are considered to be equal and constant [13].

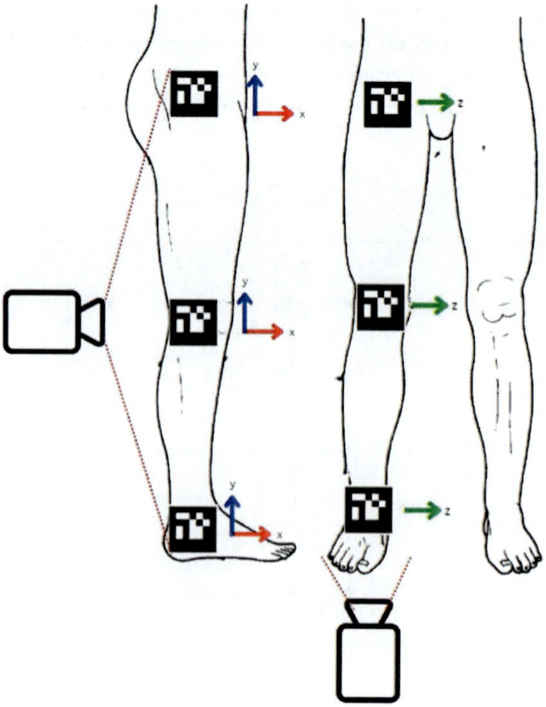

Fig. 3. Positioning of Aruco Markers.

AruCo markers are placed at the joint points as seen in Fig. 3. There are 2 Aruco markers at each joint for -dimensional linear acceleration measurement. 3-dimensional linear acceleration measurement can be conducted for each joint with 2 cameras as a result. A total of 12 AruCo markers are used at 6 joints on 2 legs.

Image Processing Algorithm. Image processing software has developed using the OpenCV library to work with 2 cameras. The algorithm calculates the markers center positions and marker edge lengths, afterwards uses them to calculate linear velocity and linear acceleration. The flow diagram of the image processing algorithm is as seen in Fig. 4. Linear velocity and linear acceleration calculation for vertical (Y) and horizontal (X) axes are as seen in Eq. 1 and Eq. 2 after the position and edge length are found in pixels.

$$\dot{X}[n] = \frac{x[n] - x[n-1]}{\tau} \times l \times \frac{1}{\rho[n]} \tag{1}$$

$$\ddot{X}[n] = \frac{\dot{x}[n] - \dot{x}[n-1]}{\tau} \tag{2}$$

$x[n]$ corresponds the center point of the marker in pixels, τ corresponds the sampling time in seconds, $\rho[n]$ corresponds the length of marker's edge in pixels and l corresponds the real length of marker's edge in meters in Eq. 1 which calculates the linear velocity of the center of the Aruco Marker. The linear acceleration can be calculated with similar method as seen in the Eq. 2.

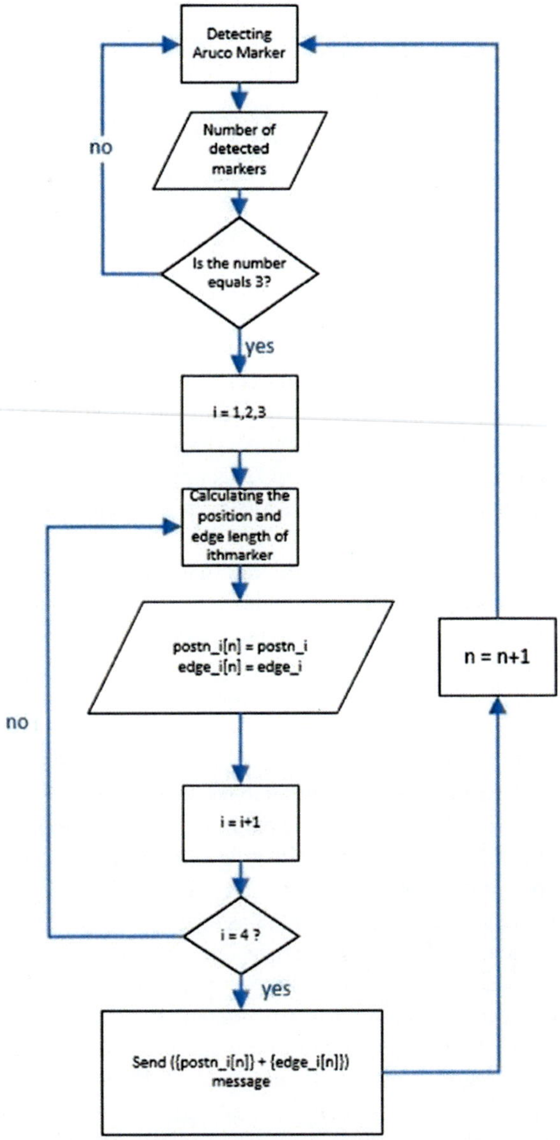

Fig. 4. The algorithm to calculate the center position and edge length of Aruco Marker.

3 IoT and Server Infrastructure

Gait analysis can be considered as a indoor object tracking problem and a data-driven analyze method. Internet of things solutions meets the fundamental requirements of such applications [14]. Therefore, it is necessary and important to collect, store, process and monitor sensor and image processing data in data-driven analyze methods like gait analysis. It is obvious that a reliable gait analysis system that uses sensor and visual data should have a communication and data storage infrastructure provides following features.

- Data loss and communication delay should be minimal during the process.
- Collected data should be able to be stored for a long time without data loss.
- Users should be able to access data easily and the system should provide a user-friendly interface to medical experts.
- The server should be low-power, portable, and accessible.

These features can be met in a internet of things infrastructure with machine- to-machine communication and database access. Therefore, main IoT communication protocol of this infrastructure has chosen as Message-Queuing-Telemetry- Transport (MQTT) protocol. The sensors and image processing software in the system are be able to send data to the server by subscribing to different topics using MQTT protocol independently from each other. Microcontrollers with wireless communication feature and the image processing software are using MQTT communication protocol to minimize data loss. The handshake feature in the MQTT protocol can significantly reduce data loss.

The data received from both the camera and the sensors are sent to the servers in JSON message format with MQTT communication. Key-value parsing has conducted for a JSON message obtained from the camera and the values obtained are seen in Table 1. The data sent from the camera includes the coordinates of marker's center point and acceleration values, as well as the time stamp of the moment the message was sent as can be seen from the Table 1.

Figure 5 shows the IoT and server infrastructure diagram of the system. MQTT communication has used between the gait analysis server, the sensor groups and image processing software as can be seen from the diagram. MQTT communication within the server is used between the database and the interface. The gait analysis server creates its own wireless communication network which enables all devices to access server's network and reach users to interface and database easily.

The industrial internet of things server design made by Yapakçı in 2022 is taken as an example in the server architecture [15]. ThingsBoard, Node- Red and Mosquitto software in this architecture are similarly utilized, and the ability of the server to create its own wireless network has been added to this architecture. The gait analysis server also acts as a DHCP server and assigns IP addresses to the devices connected. Thus the server shares internet to its own local network while the server is connected to internet with its Ethernet port. Therefore, users who access the gait analysis system server can not only access the system interface and database, but also stay connected to the internet.

Table 1. The parsed JSON message from image processing output.

Key	Value
AccX13	7.44
AccX23	3.72
AccX33	1.86
AccY13	−9.81
AccY23	−9.81
AccY33	−4.23
Timestamp3	2023-07-19 14:45:57.699257
CenterX13	336
CenterY13	173
CenterX23	339
CenterY23	314
CenterX33	336
CenterY33	392

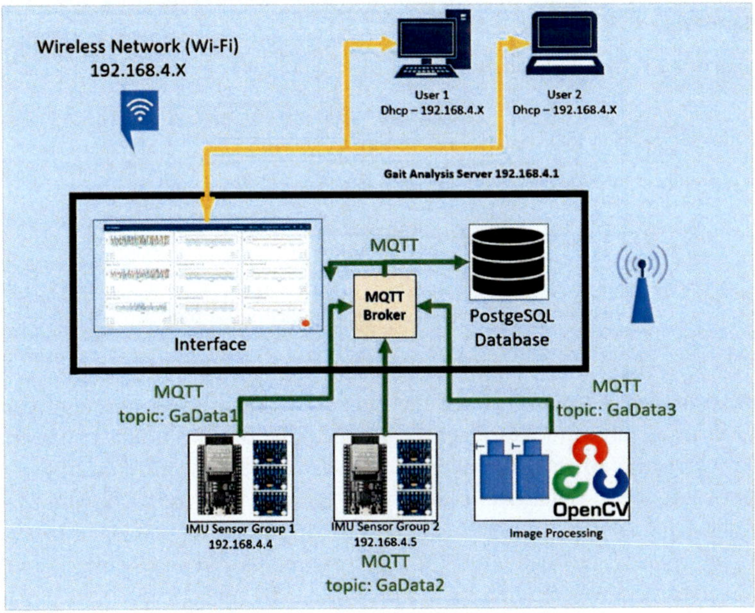

Fig. 5. IoT and server infrastructure diagram.

The interface monitors both IMU and image processing data while offers users easy and accessible data tracking. Users can also access historical data through the same interface.

A data synchronization and position estimation algorithm has been developed in order to bring together the IMU and image processing data that can be stored in the database.

4 Data Synchronization and Pose Estimation

It has been explained that 3D linear acceleration data from the accelerometer, 3D angular velocity data from the gyroscope and 3D linear acceleration data from the image processing software have obtained and stored. However, these data should be synchronized and angular position estimation should be calculated for each joint with appropriate filter structures in order to obtain meaningful gait cycle results.

It is planned to filter the linear acceleration data obtained from the camera and the linear acceleration data obtained from the accelerometer together, thus obtaining a single linear acceleration value. It is aimed to solve the following problems with this method.

- Reducing the effects of communication delays and data losses caused by wireless communication and MQTT protocol,
- Reset the average value bias from the IMU sensor's pose posture and gravitational acceleration.

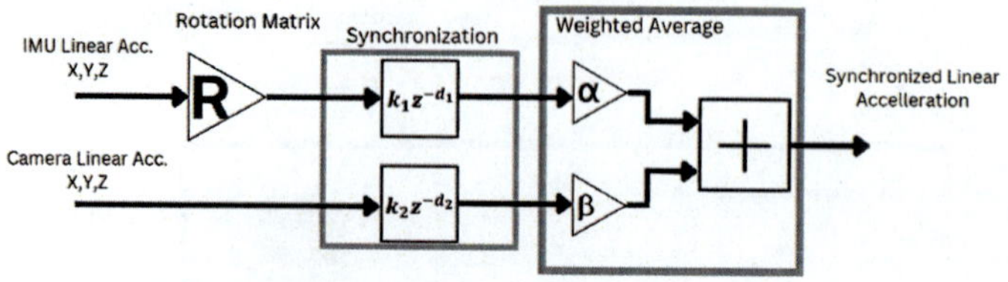

Fig. 6. Joint linear acceleration calculation process.

Figure 6 shows the joint linear acceleration calculation process from the camera and IMU linear acceleration measurements. Accordingly, the IMU data is first multiplied by a rotation matrix to reset the average value trends due to the pose posture of the IMU sensor and the gravitational acceleration. The rotation matrix for the $Z - Y - X$ Euler angles is as seen in Eq. 3. Seen here α, β, and γ are the angles of rotation about the Z, Y and X axes, respectively [16]. The rotation matrix is calculated to rotate 90 degrees counterclockwise around the z-axis while IMU sensors and AruCo markers are positioned in the body properly.

$$\mathbf{R} = \begin{bmatrix} c\alpha c\beta & c\alpha s\beta s\gamma - s\alpha c\gamma & c\alpha s\beta c\gamma + s\alpha s\gamma \\ s\alpha c\beta & s\alpha s\beta s\gamma + c\alpha c\gamma & s\alpha s\beta c\gamma - c\alpha s\gamma \\ -s\beta & c\beta s\gamma & c\beta c\gamma \end{bmatrix} \tag{3}$$

The camera and sensor data operating at different sampling times must be synchronized after applying the rotation matrix to the IMU data. The synchronization of camera and IMU linear acceleration measurements was solved in a study by Bleser and Stricker in 2009, by keeping device data operating at different sampling intervals in a message buffer [17]. Since the sensor groups and the image processing software are subscribed to the server independently of each other, the option to keep them in the buffer is not applied in this system.

There are also uncertain communication delays due to wireless communication and handshake feature in MQTT protocol. According to Lee, communication delays at the zeroth quality of service level (QoS) in wireless communications using the MQTT protocol can vary between 0.4 s and 0.7 s. While these delay amounts vary between 0.5 and 0.8 s when QoS is 1, they can vary between 0.6 seconds and 1 second at the when QoS ins 2. [18]. These delay amounts can cover the sampling periods of both camera and sensor groups in the system. Moreover, the high message publish frequency in the systems can also slow down the communication.

This data synchronization problem in the system has been solved by adding a timestamp to the sent data. Camera and sensor data can be synchronized by shifting on the sample axis according to the timestamps in each message as can be seen from Table 1. This synchronization corresponds to the synchronization block shown in Fig. 7. The synchronization is performed by setting the delay parameters d_1 and d_2 for each data group by the user.

The camera and IMU linear acceleration values are combined with the weighted average method at the end of the joint linear acceleration calculation process of the camera and IMU in Fig. 7. The inclusion of the camera and IMU structures in the common linear acceleration values can be adjusted by adjusting the α and β parameters.

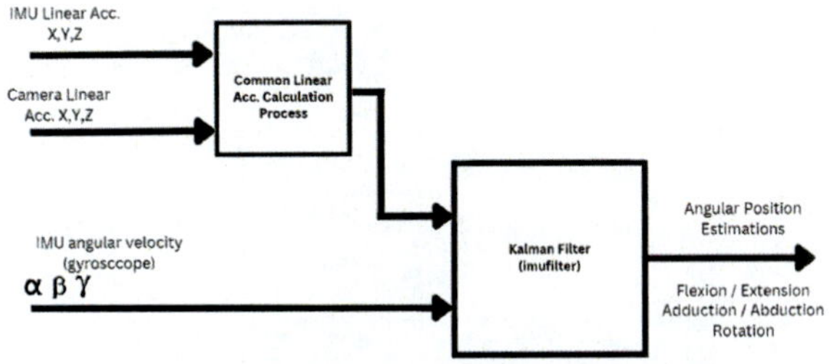

Fig. 7. The estimation process with Kalman filtering.

Figure 7 shows the joint position estimation process that after synchronization. The synchronized linear accelerations are inserted into the Kalman filter together with the angular velocity results obtained from the gyroscope, and as a result, the estimation values of flexion, extension, abduction, adduction and rotation movements in degrees are obtained.

5 Application

Figure 8 shows the measurement made with the developed gait analysis system on the treadmill with a speed of 1 m/s. Data were collected from the right leg sensor group and right leg cameras for approximately 2 min. during this measurement process. Detected AruCo markers are seen at the joint points. The synchronized linear acceleration values for the joint point in the knee with the data collected from the IMU and camera are as in Fig. 9 when $d_1 = 2$ and $d_2 = 0$ are selected.

It is observed that the phases match between the linear acceleration values obtained from the camera and the IMU with the synchronization. However, it is obvious that the amplitudes of the linear accelerations obtained are different at some points. The weighted average comparison of the acceleration value for the joint point in the knee is as seen in Fig. 10 while $\alpha = 0.6$ and $\beta = 0.4$.

The comparison between the joint angular position estimations and golden medical standart for the same patient for 1 gait cycle when the linear acceleration data and angular velocities applied into Kalman filter according to Fig. 9 is as seen in the Fig. 11.

The gait data defined as "Camera+IMU" was obtained for $\alpha = 0.6$ and $\beta = 0.4$ in Fig. 12. The gait data obtained without the camera effect was closer to the medical standard than the data with camera synchronization at each joint point for $\alpha = 0.6$ and $\beta = 0.4$. The results for different α and β values should also be examined in order to test the effect of camera synchronization.

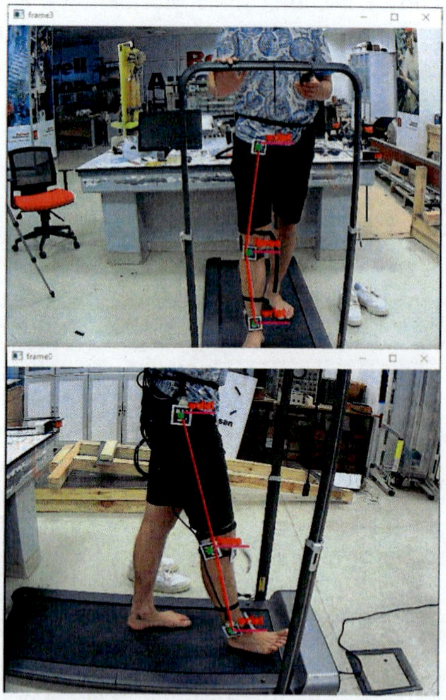

Fig. 8. Application of gait analysis system.

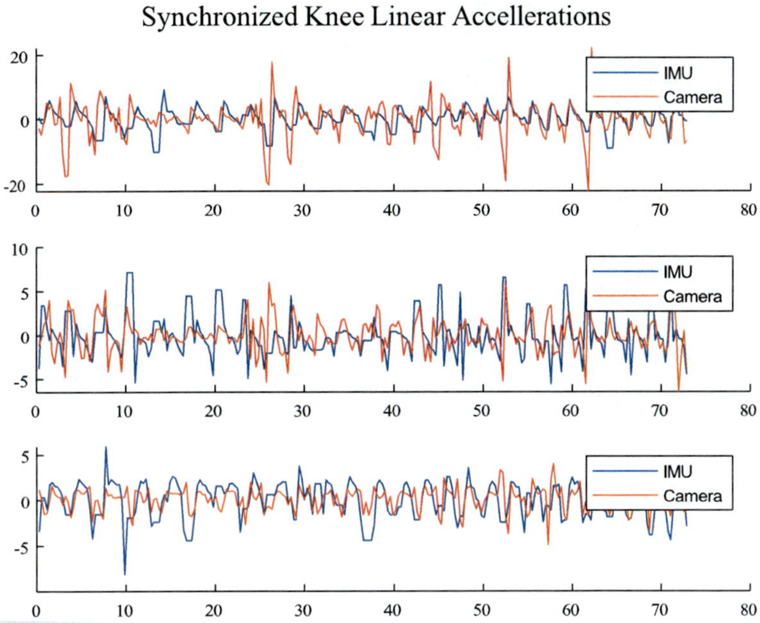

Fig. 9. Synchronized Linear accelerations from IMU and camera for while $d1 = 2$ and $d2 = 0$.

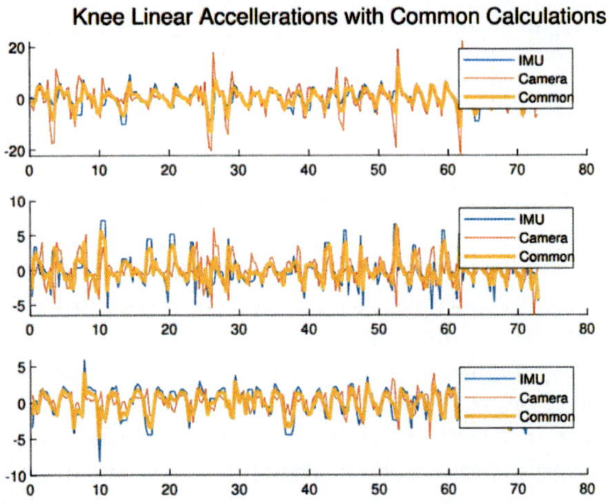

Fig. 10. Combination of accelerations for $\alpha = 0.6$ and $\beta = 0.4$.

6 Effect of Camera Synchronization

α and β values are provided to take different values between 0 and 1 in order to examine the camera effect. α is taken from 0 to 1 and β has calculated as $\beta = 1 - \alpha$. The results of 1 walking cycle for all values between 0 and 1 are as shown in Fig. 12 in this case.

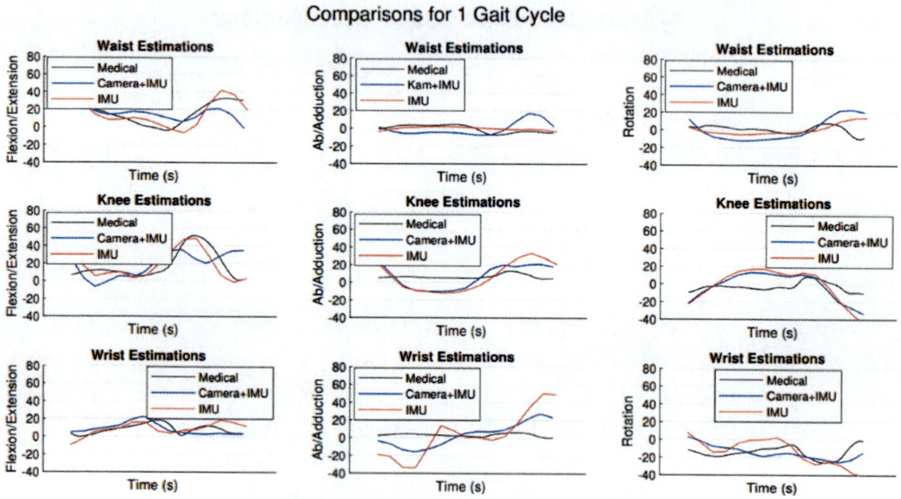

Fig. 11. The comparison of result for 1 gait cycle.

Correlation analysis has conducted between the medical standard data and the results obtained according to different α and β values for all of these values. Correlation analysis results for each joint point are as seen in Fig. 13.

It is possible to comment from Figs. 12 and 13 that the level of camera integration effects the estimated gait data in various perspectives for different joints. Figure 12 shows that both %100 and %0 levels of camera integration matches with golden standart data between an interval of degrees. However, the level of camera integration differs the gait phases and the maximum-minimum points while it also effects the rising and falling periods. The estimations for wrist joints matches the golden standart data in term of degree values while waist and knee joints matches the golden standart data in term of gait phases.

Figure 13 shows that the different % of camera integration effects the golden standart data-estimated data variously. However, it is obvious that the correlation drops as camera integration level increases for majority of joints. There are also some joint movements that include a interval of integration that increases the correlation before it drops such as wrist flexion/extension, wrist orientation, knee orientation and waist orientation.

It's also conceivable to state that the movement at waist joints are limited due to the controlled walking space of the treadmill. Therefore, the joint movements at waist joints are harder to get detected from cameras and that causes uncorrelation between golden standart data and estimated waist movements when the results get compared with other joints. It can be concluded that camera synchronization would produce more accurate gait data at waist joints in free walking applications which also have data capturing limitations. Moreover, the correlation and degree-phase match can be effected from walking speed, camera angles and IMU orientations.

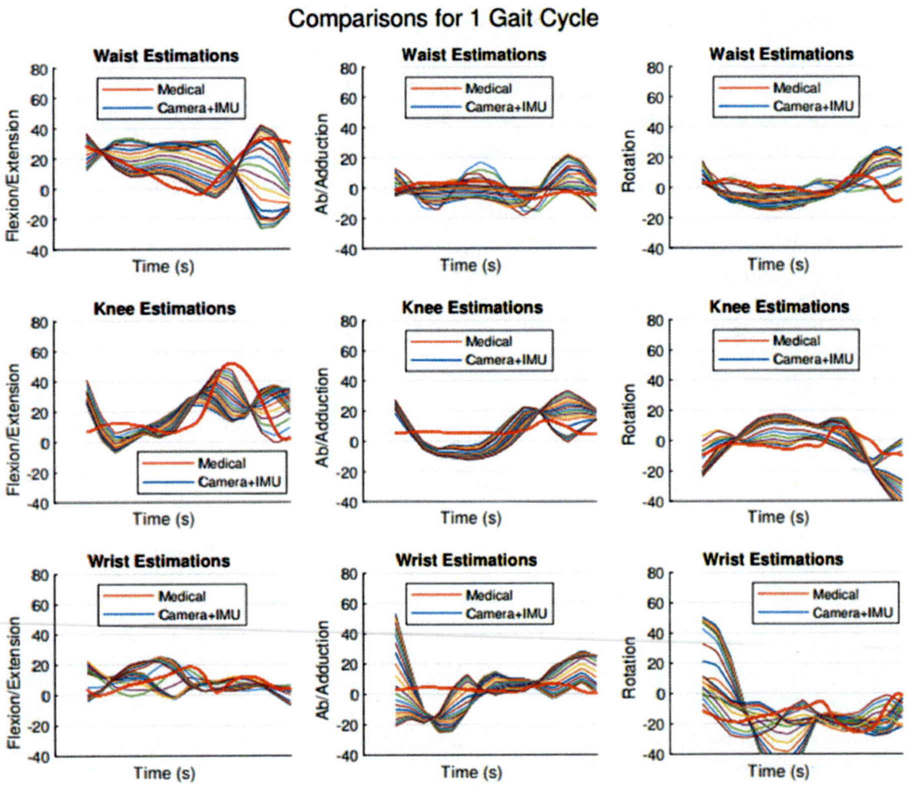

Fig. 12. Comparison of 1 gait cycles for different integration levels of camera calibration.

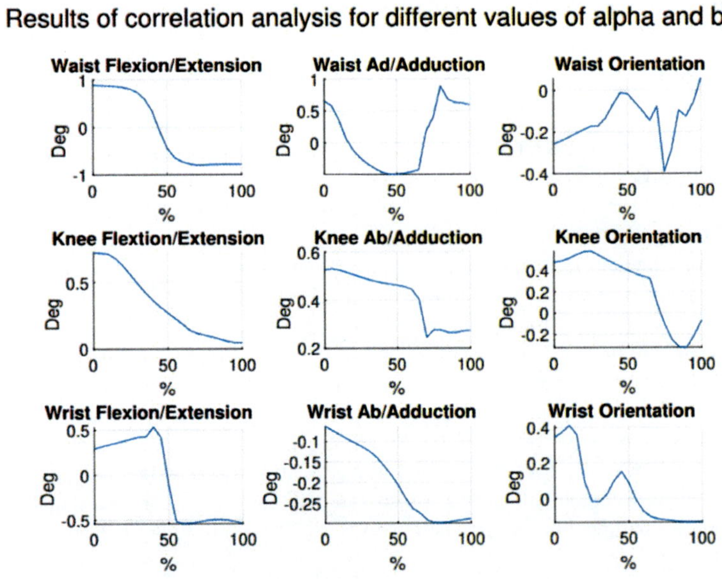

Fig. 13. Results of correlation analysis for different values of α and β.

7 Conclusion and Future Work

The gait analysis system study performed with live image processing and sensor interpretation software using Internet of Things communications and servers is explained in this paper. Live image processing and acceleration calculation algorithms, data communication diagrams are explained in detail, server structure and user interface are explained. Synchronization and estimation methods are also explained and the results are shared.

It can be said that the gait analysis system established in the study provides the following features.

- Live linear acceleration measurement with image processing,
- A developable and expandable open-source IoT and cloud infrastructure for gait analysis applications,
- Camera measurement results can overlap with the accelerometer data in phase and amplitude,
- The gait movements at the joint points of the item can be captured with both IMU data and camera-IMU synchronized data,
- Improvement of motion estimations at various joints with camera synchronization.

However, there are points to be improved and problems to be solved in the system. These can be listed as follows.

- Image processing frequency should be increased and sampling periods should be shortened.
- It should also be possible to obtain rotational movements with the camera.
- Synchronization and filtering algorithms should be improved.
- system hardware should be developed to obey the clinical standards.

The deficiencies of the developed gait analysis system will continue to be developed and its compliance with clinical standards will be increased.

References

1. Tao, W., Liu, T., Zheng, R., Feng, H.: Gait analysis using wearable sensors. Sensors **12**(2), 2255–2283 (2012)
2. Hori, K., et al.: Inertial measurement unit-based estimation of foot trajectory for clinical gait analysis. Front. Physiol. **10**, 1530 (2020)
3. Yeasin, M., Chaudhuri, S.: Development of an automated image processing system for kinematic analysis of human gait. Real-Time Imaging **6**(1), 55–67 (2000)
4. Bersamira, J.N., et al.: Human gait kinematic estimation based on joint data acquisition and analysis from imu and depth-sensing camera. In: 2019 IEEE 11th International Conference on Humanoid, Nanotechnology, Information Technology, Communication and Control, Environment, and Management (HNICEM), pp. 1–6. IEEE, November 2019
5. Young, F., Mason, R., Morris, R. E., Stuart, S., Godfrey, A. (2023). IoT-enabled gait assessment: the next step for habitual monitoring. Sensors **23**(8), 4100
6. Zhang, Q., et al.: Wearable triboelectric sensors enabled gait analysis and waist motion capture for IoT-based smart healthcare applications. Adv. Sci. **9**(4), 2103694 (2022)

7. Young, F., Mason, R., Morris, R., Stuart, S., Godfrey, A.: Internet-of-Things-Enabled Markerless Running Gait Assessment from a Single Smartphone Camera. Sensors **23**(2), 696 (2023)
8. Hahm, K.S., Anthony, B.W.: In-home health monitoring using floor-based gait tracking. Internet Things **19**, 100541 (2022)
9. Stefanović, F., Caltenco, H.: A portable measurement system for the evaluation of human gait. J. Autom. Control **19**(1), 1–6 (2009)
10. Qiu, S., Liu, L., Zhao, H., Wang, Z., Jiang, Y.: MEMS inertial sensors based gait analysis for rehabilitation assessment via multi-sensor fusion. Micromachines **9**(9), 442 (2018)
11. Whittle, M.W.: Gait analysis: an introduction. Butterworth-Heinemann (2014)
12. Garrido-Jurado, S., Muñoz-Salinas, R., Madrid-Cuevas, F. J., Marín-Jiménez, M.J.: Automatic generation and detection of highly reliable fiducial markers under occlusion. Pattern Recogn. **47**(6), 2280-2292 (2014)
13. Sarmadi, H., Muñoz-Salinas, R., Berbís, M.A., Medina-Carnicer, R.J.I.A.: Simultaneous multi-view camera pose estimation and object tracking with squared planar markers. IEEE Access **7**, 22927–22940 (2019)
14. Yelamarthi, K., Aman, M.S., Abdelgawad, A.: An application-driven modular IoT architecture. Wireless Communications and Mobile Computing (2017)
15. Yapakçı, B., Ayvaz, B., Ergenç, A.F.: Endüstriyel Nesnelerin İnterneti Sunucusu Tasarımı, Geliştirilmesi ve Uygulaması Design, Development and Implementation of a New Industrial Internet of Things Server
16. Lee, J.K., Park, E.J., Robinovitch, S.N.: Estimation of attitude and external acceleration using inertial sensor measurement during various dynamic conditions. IEEE Trans. Instrumentation Measurement **61**(8), 2262–2273 (2012)
17. Bleser, G., Stricker, D.: Advanced tracking through efficient image processing and visual–inertial sensor fusion. Comput. Graph. **33**(1), 59–72 (2009)
18. Lee, S., Kim, H., Hong, D. K., Ju, H.: Correlation analysis of MQTT loss and delay according to QoS level. In: The International Conference on Information Networking 2013 (ICOIN), pp. 714–717. IEEE, January 2013

Reducing Patient Waiting Time in Ultrasonography Using Simulation and IoT Application

İlkay Saraçoğlu[1](✉) and Çağrı Serdar Elgörmüş[2]

[1] Department of Industrial Engineering, Haliç University, Eyüpsultan, İstanbul, Turkey
ilkays@sbbdanismanlik.com

[2] Department of Emergency, Faculty of Medicine, Istanbul Atlas University, Istanbul, Turkey

Abstract. In this study, the ultrasound (US) department of a private hospital located in the most densely populated region of Istanbul is discussed. Patients can come to the US Department randomly from outpatient clinic, emergency, or inpatient departments. The time between patients' arrival at the US department varies according to hours. The types and durations of US procedures also differ in patients who come to the US department from different units. The aim of the study is to minimize the waiting time in the US department and the total time spent in the US according to the units they come from and the type of procedure to be performed. By analyzing the current situation, the performance indicators of the US department of the hospital, the average waiting time of the patients, the utilization rates of the doctors and the time spent by the patient in the US were examined. The system was modeled using the simulation method and the current state performance criteria were calculated. With the changes to be made in IoT applications and alternative system design, it is aimed to minimize the waiting time and the time spent by the patients in the system.

Keywords: Ultrasound · Simulation · IoT · Health Services · Patient Waiting Time

1 Introduction

Patient waiting times are one of the most important performance indicators of hospitals [1, 2]. Ultrasound has an important role in the diagnosis of many diseases and in the treatment of some diseases with interventional methods. Ultrasound devices are very expensive and in limited supply. Their efficient use is of great importance in controlling more patients, preventing patient victimization by reducing waiting times and efficiently using the number of doctors. Therefore, this study is an attempt to increase efficiency by taking data from the ultrasound department of a private hospital with the highest population density in Istanbul.

Sound waves have several uses within the domains of technology and medicine. Ultrasound is a medical imaging technique that utilizes sound waves to generate visual representations of the internal structures and organs within the body. Ultrasound is

A. Souri and S. Bendak (Eds.): IoTHIC 2023, ECPSCI 8, pp. 178–189, 2024.
https://doi.org/10.1007/978-3-031-52787-6_14

applied in the form of direct contact of a special device to the area to be imaged. Ultrasonography is one of the most widely used imaging techniques in the field of medicine, which is developed for diagnosing diseases related to these regions by imaging the parts of the body that cannot be seen with the naked eye and cannot be accessed by endoscopy, and to observe changes and developments. It offers diagnosis and treatment opportunities in many areas, especially the organs in the abdominal cavity, breast screening and pregnancy follow-up. The main areas where ultrasound is used can be specified as follows:

- Screenings for the baby's health status in pregnant women
- Detection of possible malfunctions in the working order of the heart
- Investigation of various infections
- Detection of gallstones and diseases
- Investigation of tumors in breast and soft tissues
- Investigations on muscle diseases
- Investigation of prostate and genital area diseases
- Ensuring imaging in interventions with needles in cyst and biopsy treatments
- Investigation of thyroid gland diseases.

In this study, the problem of patient arrivals in the ultrasound department, which is the most problematic department of a private hospital located in one of the most densely populated areas, is addressed. This paper constructs a simulation methodology to evaluate the real system and offer new system by using the IoT solutions to improve the patient waiting time. The main contribution of this paper is to show the variability in patient arrivals and waiting times that may occur with the widespread use of IoT applications in the ultrasound department.

The remainder of this paper is organized as follows: Sect. 2 presents the literature review. Section 3 defines the methodology, which includes data collection, simulation model, and results. Finally, conclusions and recommendations are presented in Sect. 4.

2 Literature Review

Since the aim of the study is to evaluate the performance of the real system using simulation method and to improve the system with IoT solutions, the first research in the literature review focused on the applications of simulation method in hospitals. Due to stochastic processes such as patient arrival times and service times in the healthcare sector, researchers have mostly conducted simulation-based studies [3]. It is seen that simulation in the health sector is mostly done for the emergency department. They examined the emergency department of a hospital using ARIS and Arena simulation programs for the emergency department [4]. The aim of their study was to use simulation modeling to reduce the waiting time of patients and increase the efficiency of doctors while evaluating the emergency department. [5] conducted a study on evaluating the waiting time of patients by simulation modeling in the emergency department. [6] improved the emergency department with a new triage team using simulation method. [7, 8] tried to reduce patient waiting time by simulating different scenarios for the emergency department.

This article focuses on the ultrasound department, which is one of the problematic departments as a result of the interview with the hospital management A literature review was conducted on the waiting times of patients in the radiology department and the study of [1] was found. As a result of the literature review, it was pointed out that the studies on the radiology department were statistically insufficient. In the literature review conducted in line with this study, very few studies on reducing the waiting time of patients in the Ultrasound department were found. For the radiology department [9], they tried to show how to model with simulation. [3] developed a simulation model that evaluates the performance of the ultrasound department if different appointment scheduling policies are followed. With Industry 4.0, technological developments are also followed in the health sector. [10] states that Healthcare 4.0 includes Industry 4.0 processes such as IoT, AI, cloud computing. In doing so, Healthcare 4.0 processes used to access data will be validated using statistical simulation and optimization methods and algorithms. In order to show the effect of the use of the wearable breast ultrasound device developed by [11, 12] on the waiting times of patients, the current situation analysis and the situation in which breast ultrasound can be easily applied by the patient herself without coming to the ultrasound department were compared in this study.

3 Methodology

3.1 Data Collection

In this study, the data of the patients who were treated in the US department of the hospital in question between January 2021 and August 2023 were analyzed. Patients come to the polyclinic departments of the hospital by appointment. As a result of the examination, the doctor can refer the patient to the US department by filling out the request form when US procedure is required. In line with this request, the patient goes to the US department to have the procedures performed and after receiving the result report, he/she goes back to the doctor where he/she was examined and shows the result report. Therefore, the arrival of patients to the US department is random. The requested US procedure times of the incoming patients also differ from each other according to the type of procedure. Figure 1 shows the number of patients coming to the US department on an hourly basis on weekends and weekdays.

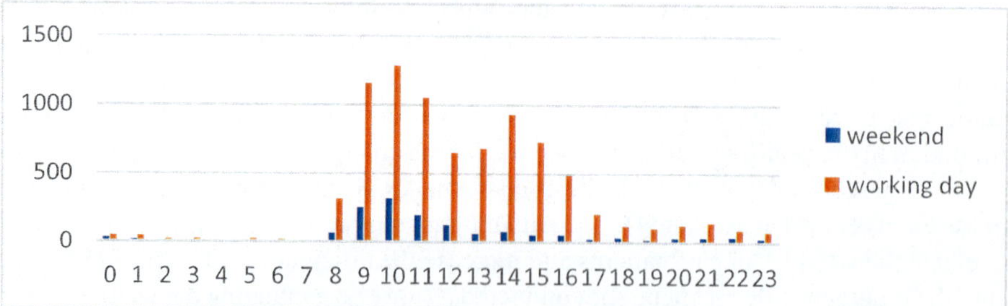

Fig. 1. Hourly served patients number according to the working day and weekend

Figure 2 shows the number of patients coming to the US department on hourly basis. Figure 3 shows the number of patients coming to the US department by years and months.

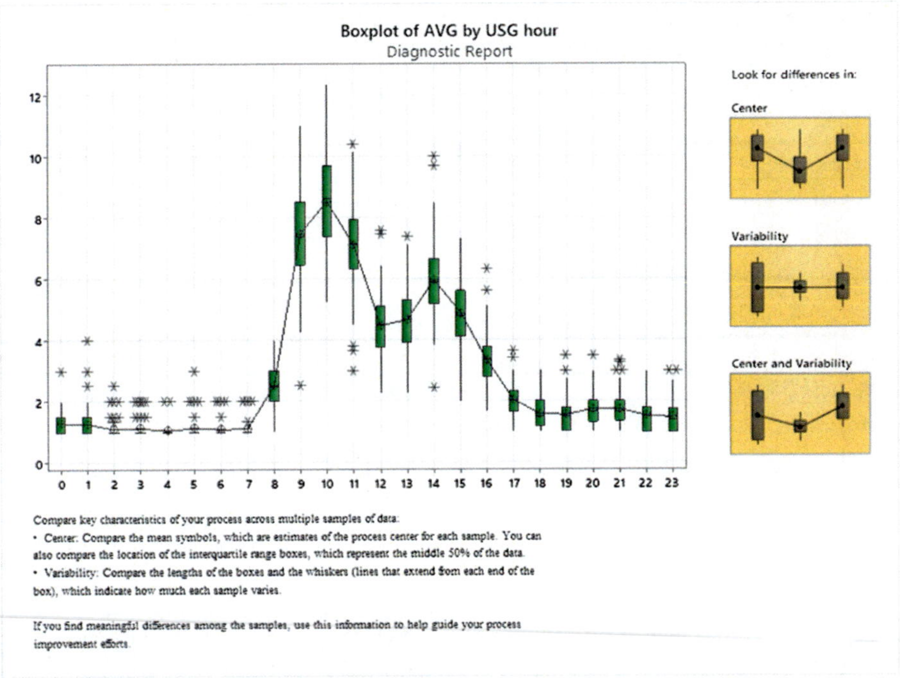

Fig. 2. Hourly served patients number by years

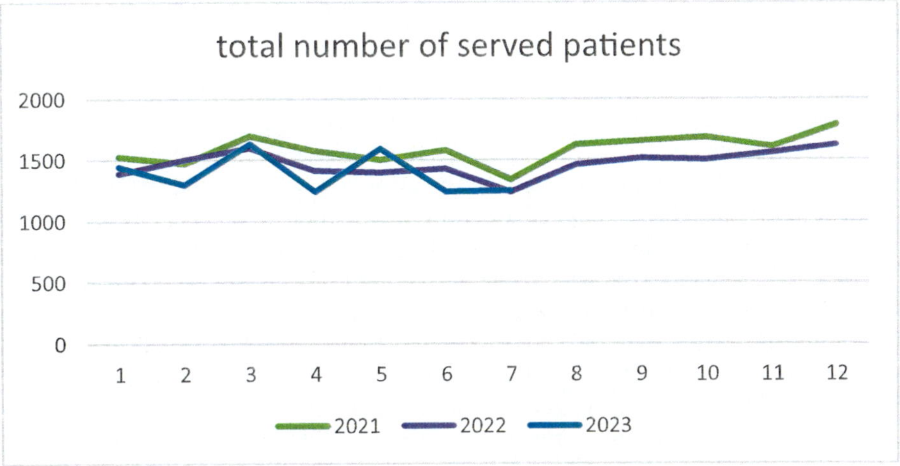

Fig. 3. Arrival patient numbers to US department

ANOVA analysis showed that there was no difference in the number of patients coming to the US department according to years and days (Fig. 4). However, a statistically significant difference is observed between hours at 95% confidence level (Fig. 5). The difference was also analyzed by Tukey analysis. According to the results of this analysis, time zones were grouped as shown in Table 1.

Analysis of Variance for years

Source	DF	Adj SS	Adj MS	F-Value	P-Value
US year	2	22.8	11.406	1.87	0.155
Error	1928	11782.1	6.111		
Total	1930	11804.9			

Analysis of Variance for days

Source	DF	Adj SS	Adj MS	F-Value	P-Value
US day	30	31.4	1.048	0.17	1.000
Error	1900	11773.5	6.197		
Total	1930	11804.9			

Fig. 4. ANOVA for years and days

Analysis of Variance for hours

Source	DF	Adj SS	Adj MS	F-Value	P-Value
US hour	23	10480	455.631	655.57	0.000
Error	1907	1325	0.695		
Total	1930	11805			

Fig. 5. ANOVA for hour

It is seen that the time interval between 10:00 and 11:00 is the time period when the highest number of patients come. After 18:00, the number of patients coming to the US department decreases. In this table, patient arrivals are shown on average. The most appropriate distribution was obtained by using Arena Input Analyzer with the chi-square test, which is the test of goodness to the distribution of the intervals between the visits of the patients to the US department. Here, as an example, the distribution of the time between arrivals of the patients who came to the US department between 10:00 and 11:00, which is the busiest time period, and the appropriate test results are given in Fig. 6. According to Fig. 6, the corresponding p-value is 0.578. This value shows that our data conforms to the Beta distribution at 90% significance level. Table 2 shows the distributions obtained by testing for all time zones.

As a result of the analysis for a period of 930 days, the most frequently performed operations in the US department were selected, and since the durations of these operations differed, a test of goodness of fit to distribution was applied for each operation. As a result of this analysis, the service time of each US type in Table 3 were found by using the Arena Input Analyzer.

Patients come to the US department randomly from the emergency department, the intensive care unit, inpatient or outpatient departments. According to the information obtained from the historical data of the hospital, 99% of the patients come from outpatient

Table 1. Grouping Information Using the Tukey Method and 95% Confidence for hours

US hour	N	Mean	Grouping								
10	93	8.522	A								
9	93	7.451		B							
11	93	7.090		B							
14	93	5.955			C						
15	93	4.884				D					
13	93	4.6680				D					
12	93	4.466				D					
16	93	3.3289					E				
8	93	2.5151						F			
17	93	2.0367							G		
20	91	1.7450							G	H	
21	93	1.7408							G	H	
18	93	1.5890								H	I
19	92	1.5621								H	I
22	89	1.5188								H	I
23	89	1.4789								H	I
0	83	1.2995								H	I
1	74	1.2797								H	I
3	60	1.1333									I
5	49	1.1327									I
7	39	1.1111									I
2	61	1.1038									I
6	48	1.0938									I
4	40	1.0500									I

clinics. As a result of the interviews with the hospital management and US doctors, it was learned that there are currently three doctors working between 9:00–18:00 on weekdays and one doctor working between 9:00–14:00. In case of an emergency, if all doctors are busy, US devices in different units are activated.

3.2 Simulation Model and Results

As a result of the interviews conducted in the US department, the patient flow chart was obtained. After the patients are examined, if the doctor refers them to the US, they first come to the US department and make the payment at the registration desk. Then, the US department secretary looks at the patient's procedure and makes referrals

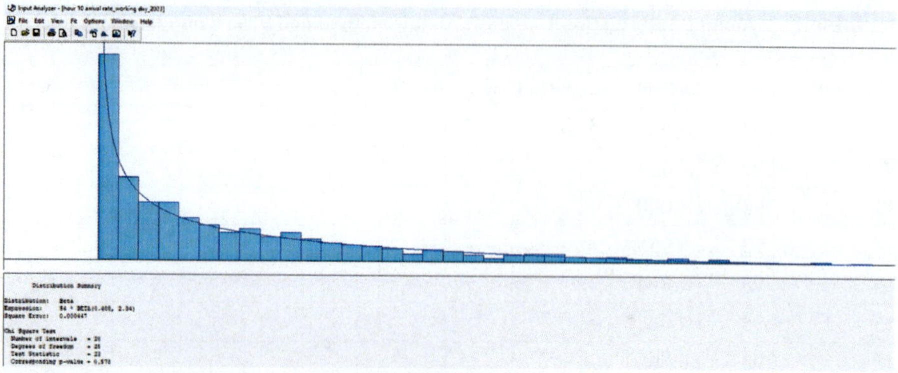

Fig. 6. Fitting a Beta distribution for between the hours of 10:00 and 11:00

Table 2. Time between arrivals of the patients

Interarrival time (hours)	Fitted Distribution	p-value
08:00–09:00	52*Beta (0.576,2.12)	0.11
09:00–10:00	−0.5 + Gamma (9.33,0.851)	0.578
10:00–11:00	54*Beta (0.488,2.34)	0.298
11:00–12:00	−0.5 + 54*Beta (0.729,3.86)	0.074
12:00–13:00	−0.5 + 28*Beta (0.669,1.48)	0.234
13:00–14:00	−0.5 + 56*Beta (0.451,1.63)	0.578
14:00–15:00	54*Beta (0.488,2.34)	0.727
15:00–16:00	Expo (11.7)	0.409
16:00–17:00	−0.5 + 61*Beta (0.636,1.95)	0.067
17:00–18:00	−0.5 + 61*Beta (0.639,1.21)	> 0.75
18:00–23:00	Expo (56.9)	> 0.75
00:00–01:00	Expo (39.6)	0.672
02:00–07:00	UNIF (1,358)	> 0.75

according to the availability of the doctors according to whether preliminary preparation is required. The patient starts the US procedure with whichever doctor is available. There are four examination rooms in the US department, each room has one doctor, one assistant and one US device. The assistant assists the doctor in preparing the patient, taking voice recordings on the computer, and preparing the report. After the US procedure is completed, the patient returns to the examination room to show the report. If the patient's procedure is abdominal US and urinary system, it is expected that the patient will be urinary tight.

Table 3. Processing times for US type patients

US type	Process Time Distribution (min)	Number of patients	Percentage
Abdominal Ultrasound	9 + Expo (5.69)	14475	36.1%
Urinary System Ultrasound	9.5 + 11*Beta (0.802,1.36)	5221	13.0%
Bilateral Breast Ultrasound	UNIF (15,30)	4504	11.2%
Neck Ultrasound	9.5 + 11*Beta (0.857,1.66)	3154	7.9%
Right hip joint Ultrasound	4.5 + Expo (2.92)	3141	7.8%
Left hip joint Ultrasound	4.5 + Expo (2.92)	2517	6.3%
Superficial Tissue Ultrasound	7 + Gamma (1.33,3.63)	2467	6.1%
Thyroid Ultrasound	UNIF (5,18)	2221	5.5%
Upper Abdominal Ultrasound	5 + Gamma (1.59,3.26)	1423	3.5%
Nuchal Translucency Measurement	10 + Erlang (3.75,2)	1013	2.5%

For this preparation phase, a minimum of 5 min and a maximum of 40 min were accepted as a uniform distribution in the model in line with expert opinions. The simulation model was created in Arena 16.0 Rockwell software and created on a computer with Intel(R) Core (TM) i7-10510U CPU @ 1.80 GHz 2.30 GHz. The simulation was run for one day with 123 replications. The main objective of the study is to minimize the waiting time of the patients in the queue. Therefore, the evaluations are based on this criterion. The simulation model of the current US department is shown in Fig. 7.

According to a model of current US department in the hospital, the expected average waiting time of a patient was 45.31 min. Validation was performed to test whether the model represents the real system. As a result of the simulation model run as 123 statistically independent replications for the real system, the average waiting time of a patient was calculated as 40.15 min and the standard deviation as 29.05 min. The simulation model was compared with the real system by applying t-test at 95% confidence level. Hypotheses established for the validation test in Eq. (1, 2):

$$H_0 = E(avg.waiting\ time) = 45.31 minutes \tag{1}$$

Versus

$$H_1 = E(avg.waiting\ time) \neq 45.31 minutes \tag{2}$$

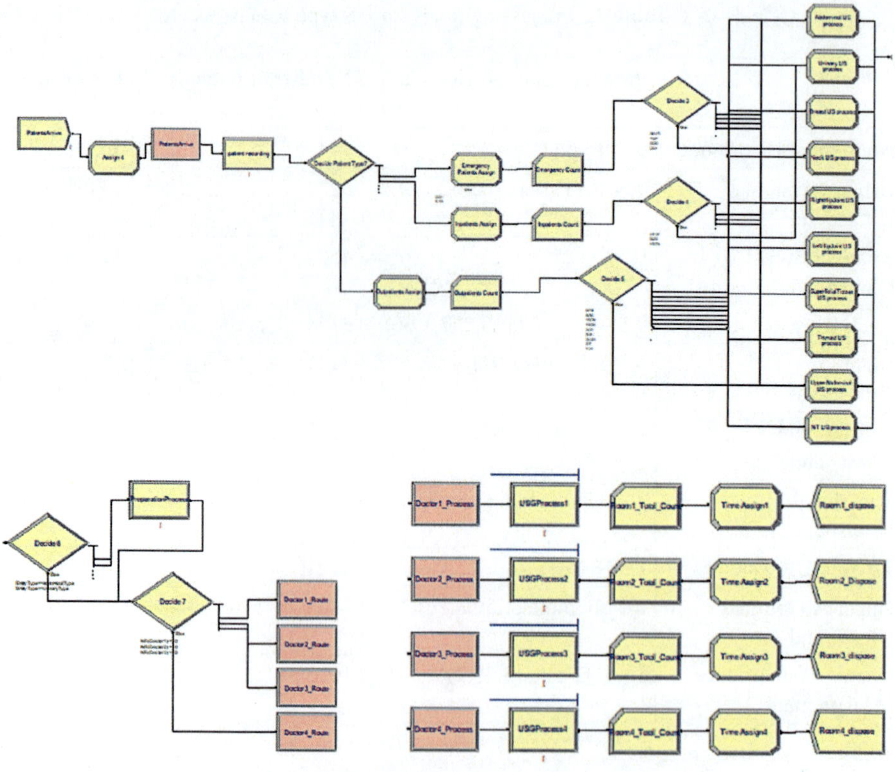

Fig. 7. Arena model for the US department in the hospital

is conducted. The significance level α and the number of samples n were chosen as 0.05 and 123, respectively. From the t table, the t value was taken as $t_{0.025,122} = 2.27$. The test statistic is calculated as Eq. (3):

$$t_0 = \frac{avg.waiting\ time - \mu_0}{S/\sqrt{n}} = \frac{40.15 - 45.31}{29.05/\sqrt{123}} = -1.97 \tag{3}$$

For the two-sided t-test, if $|t_0| > t_{\alpha/2,n-1}$, H_0 is rejected and the model is not appropriate to predict the waiting time of patients. Since $|t| = 1.97 < t_{0.025,122} = 2.27$, H_0 is accepted. The simulation model accurately represents the real system.

After testing the accuracy of the model, an alternative scenario was created for the case where it is possible to perform breast ultrasound in the patient's own comfort zone without coming to the hospital with the help of a wearable sensor, influenced by the latest technological developments. In this scenario, the breast ultrasound procedure is removed from the model. Therefore, since there is a change in the time between arrivals of the patients to the US department, the breast ultrasound was removed from the data and the time between arrivals of the patients arriving between 09:00–18:00 were recalculated. The results obtained from the second model and the results obtained from the baseline analysis were statistically tested and compared using Minitab version 21.4.1 and results are shown in Fig. 8 and Table 4.

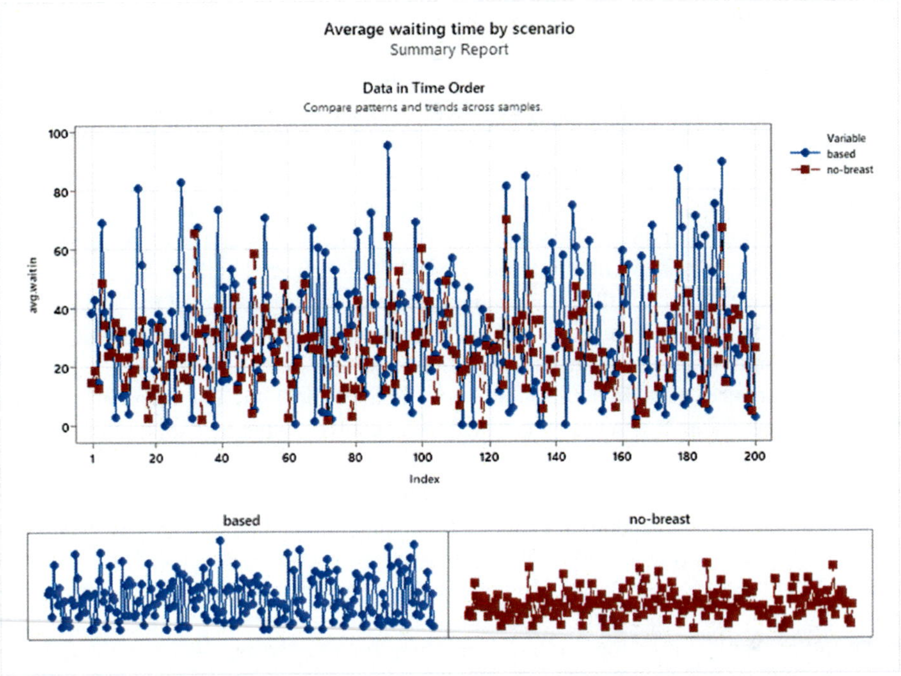

Fig. 8. Comparison of two system (based model and no-breast model)

Table 4. Results of the Analysis of Variance for compared two system

One-way ANOVA: avg waiting time versus scenario.					
Analysis of Variance					
Source	DF	Adj SS	Adj MS	F-Value	P-Value
scenario	1	3578	3578.1	6.16	0.014
Error	244	141741	580.9		
Total	245	145319			
Hypothesis:					
μ_1: replication mean of current based system					
μ_2: replication mean of no breast system					
Means					
scenario	N	Mean	StDev	95% CI	
based	123	40.15	29.05	(35.87, 44.43)	
no breast	123	32.52	17.83	(28.24, 36.80)	

4 Conclusion

In this study, as a result of the effective use of IoT in hospital processes, its effect on patient waiting time, one of the hospital performance evaluation criteria, was examined using simulation method. With the use of a wearable breast ultrasound device which was recently investigated [11], the waiting time of the patient in the US department was evaluated. While the average waiting time of the patients is 40.15 min under the current ultrasound examination process conditions, it was concluded that the expected average waiting time could be 32.52 min with the use of IoT sensor application only in the breast ultrasound process. The results showed that the average waiting time of the patient in the US department could be reduced by 19%. The analysis also showed that there could be a 39% reduction in the average number of patients waiting in the US department between 9:00–18:00 on weekdays. In addition, it is to enable the hospital management to see the expected level of improvement in the system as a result of using IoT applications within the hospital.

It was observed that abdominal ultrasound was the most common ultrasound procedure with 36.1%. Studies on this subject as IoT applications can analyze the benefits of the ultrasound department in terms of effective use of resources and cost. The evaluation of performance criteria such as the time the patient spends in the system, the number of patients waiting in the hospital, and the utilization rates of resources can be examined in the future. With simulation optimization, the number of resources can be decided in accordance with the desired goal. Different scenarios can be studied, and the system can be improved.

References

1. Olisemeke, B., Chen, Y.F., Hemming, K., Girling, A.: The effectiveness of service delivery initiatives at improving patients' waiting times in clinical radiology departments: a systematic review. J. Digit. Imaging **27**, 751–778 (2014). https://doi.org/10.1007/s10278-014-9706-z
2. Pillay, D., et al.: Hospital waiting time: the forgotten premise of healthcare service delivery? Int. J. Health Care Qual. Assur. **24**, 506–522 (2011). https://doi.org/10.1108/09526861111160553
3. Chen, P.S., Robielos, R.A.C., Palaña, P.K.V.C., Valencia, P.L.L., Chen, G.Y.H.: Scheduling patients' appointments: allocation of healthcare service using simulation optimization. J. Healthc. Eng. **6**, 259–280 (2015). https://doi.org/10.1260/2040-2295.6.2.259
4. Wang, T., Guinet, A., Belaidi, A., Besombes, B.: Modelling and simulation of emergency services with ARIS and Arena, case study: the emergency department of Saint Joseph and Saint Luc hospital. Prod. Plan. Control. **20**, 484–495 (2009). https://doi.org/10.1080/09537280902938605
5. Samaha, S., Armel, W.S., Starks, D.W.: The use of simulation to reduce the length of stay in an emergency department. In: Proceedings of the 2003 Winter Simulation Conference, vol. 2, pp. 1907–1911 (2003).https://doi.org/10.1109/wsc.2003.1261652
6. Ruohonen, T., Neittaanmäki, P., Teittinen, J.: Simulation model for improving the operation of the emergency department of special health care. In: Proceedings - Winter Simulation Conference, pp. 453–458 (2006). https://doi.org/10.1109/WSC.2006.323115
7. Gharahighehi, A., Kheirkhah, A.S., Bagheri, A., Rashidi, E.: Improving performances of the emergency department using discrete event simulation, DEA and the MADM methods. Digit. Heal. **2**, 205520761666461 (2016). https://doi.org/10.1177/2055207616664619

8. Haghighinejad, H.A., et al.: Using queuing theory and simulation modelling to reduce waiting times in an Iranian emergency department. Int. J. Commun. Based Nurs. Midwifery. **4**, 11–26 (2016)
9. Shakoor, M.: Using discrete event simulation approach to reduce waiting times in computed tomography radiology department. World Acad. Sci. Eng. Technol. Int. J. Ind. Manuf. Eng. **9**, 177–181 (2015)
10. Kumar, A., Krishnamurthi, R., Nayyar, A., Sharma, K., Grover, V., Hossain, E.: A novel smart healthcare design, simulation, and implementation using healthcare 4.0 processes. IEEE Access **8**, 118433–118471 (2020). https://doi.org/10.1109/ACCESS.2020.3004790
11. Du, W., et al.: Conformable ultrasound breast patch for deep tissue scanning and imaging. Sci. Adv. **9**, eadh5325 (2023). https://doi.org/10.1126/sciadv.adh5325
12. Luo, Y., et al.: Technology roadmap for flexible sensors. ACS Nano **17**, 5211–5295 (2023). https://doi.org/10.1021/acsnano.2c12606

Author Index

A. Souri and S. Bendak (Eds.): IoTHIC 2023, ECPSCI 8, p. 191, 2024.
https://doi.org/10.1007/978-3-031-52787-6